Polycystic Ovary Syndrome - Symptoms, Causes and Treatment

Edited by Zhengchao Wang

Published in London, United Kingdom

Polycystic Ovary Syndrome - Symptoms, Causes and Treatment
http://dx.doi.org/10.5772/intechopen.107755
Edited by Zhengchao Wang

Contributors
Adity Paul, Anđelka Radojčić Badovinac, Bogdan Morosan, Claudia Mehedintu, Cristina Gladys Al Jashi, Gunasekaran Ramanathan, Edu Antoine, Isam Al Jashi, Kritee Niroula, Lisa Vizza, Lisley Konar, Madan Pandey, Manshi Kumari, Mihaela Plotogea, Miruna Tanase, Neda Smiljan Severinski, Rana Alhamdan, Rituparna Das, Subrat Panda, Surya Prakash Goud Ponnam, Ulla Marton

First published in London, United Kingdom, 2024 by IntechOpen
IntechOpen is the global imprint of INTECHOPEN LIMITED, registered in England and Wales, registration number: 11086078, 167-169 Great Portland Street, London, W1W 5PF, United Kingdom

British Library Cataloguing-in-Publication Data
A catalogue record for this book is available from the British Library

Additional hard and PDF copies can be obtained from orders@intechopen.com

Polycystic Ovary Syndrome - Symptoms, Causes and Treatment
Edited by Zhengchao Wang
p. cm.

This title is part of the Obstetrics and Gynecology Book Series, Volume 3
Topic: Reproductive and Gynecologic Health
Series Editor: Zouhair O. Amarin
Topic Editor: Courtney Marsh

Print ISBN 978-0-85014-141-2
Online ISBN 978-0-85014-142-9
eBook (PDF) ISBN 978-0-85014-143-6
ISSN 3049-706X

IntechOpen Book Series

Obstetrics and Gynecology

Volume 3

Aims and Scope of the Series

Obstetrics and Gynecology field typically covers several subspecialties that include maternal-fetal medicine, gynecologic oncology, reproductive endocrinology and subfertility, urogynecology and female pelvic reconstructive surgery, critical care medicine, complex family planning, pediatric and adolescent gynecology, menopausal and geriatric gynecology, and minimally invasive gynecologic surgery.
Apart from being diverse, obstetrics and gynecology is a challenging and demanding specialty. It combines medical and surgical skills.
The sequence of books in this series will have certain characteristics in common that will be recognized as part of the same informative multi-volume book programme.

Meet the Series Editor

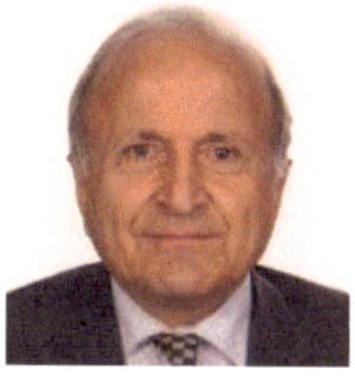

Zouhair Amarin is a Professor of Obstetrics and Gynaecology at the Jordan University of Science and Technology. He was previously a lecturer at the University of Glasgow, Scotland, a senior lecturer at the University of Nottingham, England, and the dean of the Faculty of Medicine at Mutah University, Jordan. Professor Amarin is a fellow of the Royal College of Obstetricians and Gynaecologists, and the Faculty of Public Health, London. He holds master's degrees in medical science and medical education. He is a pioneer in IVF and was the first in the world to develop microsurgical epididymis sperm aspiration for clinical use. He also discovered a surgical procedure for critical ovarian hyperstimulation syndrome. Professor Amarin has edited books, authored book chapters, and published more than 130 papers. He is the recipient of eight awards.

Meet the Volume Editor

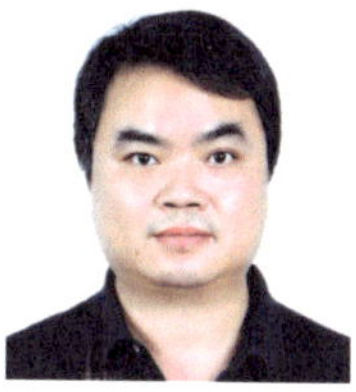

Dr. Zhengchao Wang is a full professor at the College of Life Sciences, Fujian Normal University, China. He is a principal investigator for the General Program for the National Natural Science Foundation of China and the Program for New Century Excellent Talents at the University of the Ministry of Education of China. He is also a team leader in the Fujian Provincial Key Laboratory for Developmental Biology and Neurosciences, the Key Laboratory of Optoelectronic Science and Technology for Medicine of the Ministry of Education. He obtained his Ph.D. in 2008 and has a long teaching and research career. He has published over one hundred scientific papers and over ten books as the editor in his specialty and related diseases.

Contents

Preface

Polycystic ovary syndrome (PCOS) is a major health problem. It is a heterogeneous hormone-imbalance disorder that occurs in reproductive-aged women worldwide and is characterized by hyperandrogenism, ovulatory process dysfunction, and polycystic ovaries.

PCOS is affected by various factors, and there are no unique diagnostic criteria in different regions, due to the heterogeneity of clinical manifestations and endocrine system changes of PCOS. Therefore, it is often difficult to accurately diagnose women with PCOS, as the signs and symptoms of PCOS can vary among individuals. Although PCOS is usually diagnosed during the early reproductive years, the precise pathogenesis of PCOS remains unclear. An increasing number of studies have demonstrated that the insulin signaling pathway has an important role in the pathophysiology of PCOS, including phosphatidylinositol 3-kinase and protein kinase B signaling, which is critically implicated in insulin resistance, androgen secretion, obesity, and follicular development. PCOS manifests as defective ovarian steroid biosynthesis and hyperandrogenemia, and 50–70% of women with PCOS exhibit insulin resistance and are hyperinsulinemic, indicating that insulin resistance and hyperinsulinism may have an important role in the pathophysiology of PCOS.

This book provides a comprehensive overview of the current state of the art in PCOS research to benefit the population of women with PCOS. I hope this book is meaningful to the clinicians who care for women with PCOS and to the researchers who investigate the complexities of this disease. We sincerely thank all the authors for their contributions to our book.

Dr. Zhengchao Wang
Provincial Key Laboratory for Developmental Biology and Neurosciences,
College of Life Sciences,
Fujian Normal University,
Fuzhou, China

Section 1

Polycystic Ovary Syndrome Symptoms

Chapter 1

Genetics and Epigenetics of Polycystic Ovary Syndrome

Surya Prakash Goud Ponnam and Adity Paul

Abstract

Polycystic ovary syndrome (PCOS) is one of the most common endocrinological and reproductive disorders in women of reproductive age with a global prevalence rate of 5–20%. It is a clinically and genetically heterogeneous disorder. There have been multiple reports from independent research groups from different ethnicities that a variety of factors, including genetics and epigenetics, significantly contribute to the etiopathogenesis of PCOS. GWAS, twin studies, and genotype-phenotype association studies have resulted in the identification of more than a dozen candidate genes/loci with PCOS. In the proposed book chapter, we aim to provide insight and discuss the role of various genetic and epigenetic elements that are responsible for PCOS globally and in India. This book chapter should serve as a reference to all the basic researchers and healthcare professionals on the genetics and epigenetics of PCOS.

Keywords: PCOS, genetics, epigenetics, prevalence, classification

1. Introduction

Stein and Leventhal were the first to describe women with amenorrhea, hirsutism, obesity, and ovaries that appeared to be polycystic in seven independent cases [1] and termed it as Stein-Leventhal syndrome which was subsequently referred to as polycystic ovary syndrome (PCOS). PCOS is a complex reproductive and endocrinological disorder in women of the reproductive age group across the globe. PCOS is characterized by the presence of hyperandrogenism (HA), ovulatory dysfunction (OD), and/or the presence of unilateral or bilateral polycystic ovarian morphology (PCOM).

PCOS is a multifactorial disorder with complex aetiopathophysiology. Several factors including genetic, epigenetic, lifestyle, nutrition, ethnicity, and environment are known to contribute to PCOS [2]. However, the quantum of each factor contributing to the overall phenotype is not yet ascertained. PCOS is one of the major causes of anovulatory infertility and these patients are predicted to have a high risk of developing endometrial cancer [3].

2. Clinical signs and symptoms

The three main clinical signs and symptoms of PCOS include hyperandrogenism (clinical/biochemical), menstrual irregularities (oligomenorrhoea, amenorrhoea, and/or followed by prolonged or heavy periods), and polycystic ovarian morphology (PCOM) [4].

Firstly, clinical hyperandrogenism presents itself as acne, hirsutism, alopecia, and acanthosis nigricans, and biological hyperandrogenism as excess of androgen production. Secondly, hormonal imbalance such as elevated levels of luteinizing hormone, disrupted ratio of luteinizing hormone to follicle-stimulating hormone (LH: FSH), increased Amh (anti-mullerian hormone) levels, etc. results in the development of cysts in the ovary and leads to irregular menstruation that includes anovulation and amenorrhea/oligomenorrhea [4], further leading to PCOS. Lastly, the PCOM refers to the presence of 12 or more follicles in the ovary with a diameter of 2–9 mm and an ovarian volume of around 10 ml or greater [5–7].

Various cardio-metabolic disorders are also associated with PCOS that include hyperlipidemia, insulin resistance, hypertension, type 2 diabetes mellitus, cardiovascular disease, etc. [8]. PCOS patients have also been reported to have increased neonatal complications such as pre-eclampsia, preterm birth, gestational diabetes, early pregnancy loss, etc. [9].

3. Prevalence

The global prevalence rate of PCOS was reported to be between 5 and 20% of women of reproductive age [10]. A study by Liu and co-workers analyzed the burden of PCOS to be approximately one and a half million globally, after analyzing the data in women of reproductive age ranging between 15 and 49 years across 194 counties [11]. The World Health Organization (2021) reported that approximately 116 million women (3.4%) suffer from PCOS globally [12]. Few independent research groups have reported different symptoms and prevalence rates of PCOS among different ethnicities [13, 14]. The wide difference in the prevalence rates across the globe is due to multiple reasons that include the different criteria being followed for diagnosis, ethnicity, time of publication, survey populations, etc. [15–20].

The prevalence rate of PCOS in India is reported to be ranging between 3.7% and 22.5% among women of the reproductive age group [19, 20]. A systematic review and meta-analysis by Bharali et al. reported the pooled prevalence of PCOS in Indian women to be 5.8% as per the NIH criteria and 10% as per the Rotterdam's criteria and AES criteria respectively [21].

4. Diagnosis and grading of the severity of PCOS

The definition and the diagnostic criteria for PCOS were initially laid down by The National Institute for Child Health and Human Development (NICHD), USA conference in the year 1990. As per this conference, diagnostic characteristics for PCOS included clinical and/or biochemical hyperandrogenism and menstrual irregularities [22]. The American Society for Reproductive Medicine (ASRM), European Society of Human Reproduction and Embryology (ESHRE) presented the Rotterdam criteria in 2003. According to this, at least two out of three criteria are mandatory (oligo-ovulation or anovulation, clinical or biochemical hyperandrogenism, and/or the presence of polycystic ovarian morphology), for a patient to be diagnosed with PCOS [23]. The Androgen Excess and PCOS Society, considered PCOS as primarily a hyperandrogenic disorder and defined PCOS as the presence of clinical and/or biochemical hyperandrogenism accompanied by either oligo-ovulation or polycystic ovarian morphology [24].

Rotterdam criteria is one of the widely accepted criteria for diagnosing PCOS. As per this classification, PCOS patients have been sub-grouped into four different phenotypes, namely, phenotype A (Frank or Classic polycystic type) with HA + OD + PCOM, phenotype B (Classic non-cystic type) with HA + OD, phenotype C (Non classic ovulatory type) with HA + PCOM, and phenotype D (Non classic mild or normo-androgenic type) with OD + PCOM symptoms [25].

5. Genetics of PCOS

The role of genetics in PCOS was first proposed by Cooper et al. on chromosomal analysis of 18 families of American origin and had reported an autosomal dominant mode of inheritance and decreased penetrance [26]. Wilroy and coworkers [27] observed that the male relatives of PCOS patients were diagnosed with oligospermia and increased LH secretion, suggesting an X-linked mode of inheritance. The same study also reported the association of PCOS with metabolic co-morbidities like diabetes mellitus, dyslipidaemia, hypertension, and arteriosclerosis [27]. An increase in the incidence of infertility, oligomenorrhea, and hirsutism in first-degree relatives of PCOS patients and an increased degree of baldness in male relatives was reported by Ferriman and Purdie [28]. Twin studies have suggested PCOS to be a polygenic disorder influenced by both intrauterine and extrauterine environmental factors [29, 30].

6. Few candidate genes associated with PCOS

To date, independent studies from different ethnicities and research groups have reported more than a dozen candidate genes/loci for PCOS. Majority of these candidate genes have been broadly classified into the six major pathways/groups. A few important genes in each category/pathway have been mentioned below:

i. Ovarian and adrenal steroidogenesis pathway (*CYP11A*, *CYP17*, *CYP19*)

ii. Gonadotropin action and regulation pathway (*LHCGR*, *AMH*, *FSHR*)

iii. Steroid hormone effects pathway (*AR*, *SHBG*)

iv. Insulin action and secretion pathway (*INS*, *INSR*, *CAPN10*)

v. Chronic inflammation pathway (*TNFA*)

vi. Energy homeostasis pathway (leptin and receptor genes, *ADIPOQ*, and *PPARG*)

6.1 *CYP11A* (cytochrome P450 family 11 subfamily A) gene

The locus for the *CYP11A* gene (Ensembl ID: ENSG00000140459) is 15q24.1. The *CYP11A* gene is approximately 20 kb in size and has 9 exons. *CYP11A* gene codes for a total of nine mRNA transcripts out of which only six codes for the functional protein. The largest transcript (ENST00000268053.11) is 1837 bp and encodes for the cholesterol side-chain cleavage enzyme (cytochrome P450scc) with 521 amino acids and an approximate molecular weight of 60 kDa.

The cholesterol side-chain cleavage enzyme (cytochrome P450scc) initiates steroidogenesis and converts cholesterol to pregnenolone. *Cyp11a* is expressed in the adrenal cortex, ovaries, testis, and placenta in humans [31]. Pathogenic mutations in the *CYP11A* gene have been reported in multiple diseases such as P450scc insufficiency, XY sex reversal and adrenal insufficiency, Adrenal hyperplasia, Adrenal hypospadias, etc. [31].

Gharani et al. [32] and Diamanti-Kandarakis and co-workers [33] reported a significant correlation between the alleles of the *CYP11A* gene with a 5′ untranslated region (UTR) consisting of repeats of a (tttta)n pentanucleotide and serum testosterone levels in PCOS patients. Wang et al. reported that the allele of (tttta)n microsatellite polymorphism in the promoter of the *CYP11A* gene has a higher frequency and is associated with increased BMI in the Chinese population with PCOS [34]. Zhang and co-workers reported that the SNP rs4077582 in *CYP11A1* is positively correlated to PCOS susceptibility and affects testosterone levels by regulating LH [35].

Pusalkar and coworkers found that variations in the promoter region of *CYP11A1* and *CYP17* were associated with testosterone levels in PCOS patients in the Indian population [36]. Further, this polymorphism was suggested as a potential molecular marker for PCOS by Reddy et al. in the South Indian population [37]. On the contrary, Gaasenbeek et al. studied the polymorphisms of the *CYP11A* promoter region in PCOS patients from the United Kingdom and Finland and found no significant correlation [38].

6.2 *CYP17* (cytochrome P450 family 17) gene

The locus for the human *CYP17* gene (Ensembl ID: ENSG00000148795) is 10q24.32. This gene codes for a total of 8 mRNA transcripts out of which five codes for a functional protein. The largest transcript (ENST00000369887.4) is 1750 bp and encodes for cytochrome P450 17α-hydroxylase protein with 508 amino acids and an approximate molecular weight of 57.4 kDa. Cytochrome P450 17α-hydroxylase enzyme is primarily located in the endoplasmic reticulum in humans and has hydroxylase and lyase activity. It converts progesterone and pregnenolone into 17-hydroxyprogesterone and 17-hydroxypregnenolone respectively and subsequently to 4-androstenedione and dehydroepiandrosterone [39].

Escobar-Morreale et al. reported an increased P450c17α activity in PCOS women with hyperandrogenism in the adrenal cortex and ovaries [40]. Two independent reports by Wickenheisser and co-workers have concluded that there is higher transactivation of *CYP17* promoter in ovarian theca cells and dysregulation in the expression of *CYP17* at the mRNA level [41, 42]. A T/C SNP in the promoter region was found to be associated with PCOS in the Caucasian and Greek populations by Carey et al. [43] and Diamanti-Kandarakis et al. [44] respectively. The *CYP17* gene is primarily responsible for the development of insulin resistance and a hyperandrogenic phenotype in PCOS patients [45, 46].

Kaur et al. reported a -34 T > C polymorphism in *CYP17A1* that was found to be associated with PCOS in the north Indian population [47]. Few studies have reported a negative correlation between *CYP17* polymorphisms and PCOS [48–51].

Besides PCOS, mutations in the *CYP17* gene have also been reported in 17-alpha-hydroxylase/17, 20-lyase deficiency, Steroid-17 alpha-hydroxylase deficiency, Pseudohermaphroditism, etc. [31].

6.3 *CYP19* (cytochrome P450 family 19) gene

The locus for the *CYP19* gene (Ensembl ID: ENSG00000137869) is 15q21. The size of this gene is approximately 70 kb and has 10 exons. *CYP19* gene codes for 19 transcripts, out of which only 12 codes for a functional protein. The largest transcript (ENST00000396402.6) codes for Aromatase (P450arom) or estrogen synthetase enzyme, which is 4403 bp and with 503 amino acids and has a molecular weight of approximately 53 kDa. The estrogen synthetase enzyme catalyzes the tranformation of the C19 testosterone androstenedione, and androgens, to the C18 estradiol, estrone and estrogens, respectively [46]. In humans, the expression of P450arom is in the bone, adipose stromal cells, ovary, placenta, and few foetal tissues [52].

Petry et al. [53] and Medeiros et al. [54] identified a deficiency of aromatase activity in patients with PCOS and hyperandrogenism in the British and Brazilian populations respectively [53, 54]. Yu et al. reported reduced *CYP19A1* expression in ovaries due to hypermethylation of its promoter region in PCOS patients from China [55]. Chen et al. reported a significant decrease in the activity of P450arom in both lean and obese women with PCOS [56]. In a multicentric study, the SNP (rs2414096) was reported to have a positive association between reduced aromatase activity, increased estradiol to testosterone ratio (E2/T), and PCOS development in Caucasian and African patients [57]. These findings were further corroborated by independent research groups in the Chinese [58] and Iranian [59] populations. Few studies have reported that a tetranucleotide repeat (TTTA)*n* in the *CYP19* gene with short alleles results in the inhibition of the aromatase activity and hyperandrogenism along with a high LH: FSH ratio [60, 61].

Ashraf et al. reported a SNP (rs2414096) of the *CYP19* gene to be associated the PCOS susceptibility and hyperandrogenism in patients from Kashmir, India [62].

6.4 *LHCGR* (luteinizing hormone/choriogonadotropin receptor) gene

The locus for the *LHCGR* gene (ENSG00000138039) is on chromosome 2p16.3 and has a size of approximately 80kbp. This gene codes for a total of six mRNA transcripts, out of which only five code for the functional protein, luteinizing hormone (LH)/ choriogonadotropin receptor. The largest transcript (ENST00000294954.12) is 3076 bp with 699 amino acids with an approximate molecular weight of 33 kDa.

The *LHCGR* gene, which is crucial for ovulation in response to the mid-cycle LH surge, is mostly expressed in the granulosa cells of preovulatory follicles in females [63]. The luteinizing hormone is a member of the G protein-coupled receptors (GPCR) subfamily N and is characterized by the presence of a large N-terminal extracellular domain with leucine-rich repeats (LRR).

Elevated LH levels are a common characteristic in PCOS patients, and are related to anovulation, as luteinizing hormone has a negative effect on the development of eggs [64]. Furui et al. reported two missense pathogenic mutations (Trp8Arg and Ilg15Thr) in the gene coding for the beta-subunit of the luteinizing hormone in PCOS patients [65]. On the contrary, a multinational and multicentric study by Nilsson et al. reported these changes in the normal population also [66]. Takahashi and co-workers reported many SNPs in the promoter site of the *LH* gene that were common to patients with PCOS and other ovulatory disorders [67]. GWAS studies have identified the 2p16.3 region containing *LHCGR* loci to be associated with PCOS in Han Chinese [68] and European populations [69]. An SNP (rs2293275) that induces an amino acid substitution (S312N) was reported in the Sardinian population with PCOS [70].

Thathapudi and co-workers reported the SNP (rs2293275) in the *LHCGR* gene to be associated with PCOS from Southern India [71]. Singh et al. suggested that a mutant allele (C) of rs12470652 and mutant genotype (AA) and mutant allele (A) of rs2293275 conferred a high risk of PCOS progression in the North Indian population [72].

Genetic analysis of 150 PCOS families of European and Caribbean origin for pathogenic mutations, in a total of 37 potential candidate genes, resulted in no significant correlation between the LH gene and PCOS [73].

6.5 *FSHR* (follicle-stimulating hormone receptor) gene

The locus for the *FSHR* gene (ENSG00000170820) is 2p21 and it is approximately 54 kbp in size. This gene codes for a total of five mRNA transcripts, out of which only three code for the functional protein- follicle-stimulating hormone (FSH). The largest transcript (ENST00000406846.7) is 2762 bp with 695 amino acids with an approximate molecular weight of 30 kDa. FSH promotes oogenesis, follicle development, and gametogenesis, which results in follicular maturation and granulosa cell proliferation [74].

Mutations in *FSHR* gene have been associated with ovarian hyperstimulation syndrome, ovarian cancer, premature ovarian insufficiency with resistant ovary syndrome, etc. Hypogonadotropic hypogonadism is caused by an inactivating mutation in the *FSHR* gene, which also causes arrests of the preantral stage of follicle development [75].

GWAS study in Han Chinese population by Shi et al. reported the association of the *FSHR* gene with PCOS [76]. Two SNPs, Thr307Ala and Asn680Ser in exon 10 of the *FSHR* gene have been found to be associated with PCOS from Italian [77] and South Korean populations [78]. While the SNP (rs2268361) was reported to be associated with PCOS in the Chinese population [79] it was not in the Dutch population [80].

6.6 *AMH* (anti-Mullerian hormone) gene

The locus for the *AMH* gene (ENSG00000104899) is 19p13.3. *AMH* gene codes for a total of three transcripts out of which only one transcript (ENST00000221496.5) encodes the functional protein-Anti-mullerian hormone (AMH). The size of the gene is 2.8 kbp with 5 exons. The AMH protein is a homo-dimeric precursor protein and has a molecular weight of approximately 140 kDa. The two-polypeptide chains contain a large N-terminal prodomain and a small C-terminal mature domain. The Sertoli and granulosa cells contain the major transcription initiation site, located 10 bp upstream of the ATG codon.

Amh protein has been found to suppress the release of estradiol (E2) and limit the development of ovarian follicles in response to serum FSH in the cells [81]. It regulates the early change from primordial follicles that are at rest, to developing follicles in females. Studies have reported that $AMH^{-/+}$gene null mice recruit more primordial follicles as compared to wild-type mice but also show an early depletion of their primordial follicles stock [82]. The primary pathophysiologic circumstance for the start of PCOS is follicular arrest, which is caused by Amh's interference with follicular development and recruitment. Amh also suppresses FSH-induced aromatase activity, which promotes the development of other PCOS-related clinical symptoms such as excess androgen and insulin resistance [83].

Zheng et al. reported that *AMH* gene polymorphism (rs10407022) is linked to insulin resistance in PCOS patients from China [84]. An unbiased WGS analysis of 80 PCOS patients by Gorsic et al. resulted in identifying a total of 24 rare variants in patients of European ancestry [85].

Kevenaar and co-workers reported that genetic variants in the *AMH* and *AMHR2* genes did not influence PCOS susceptibility in Dutch Caucasian patients, however, they found that AMH Ile^{49}Ser polymorphism had a positive correlation with follicle number and androgen levels [86].

6.7 *AR* (androgen receptor) gene

The locus for the *AR* gene (ENSG00000169083) is Xq12 and it has a size of 90 kbp. This gene has a total of eight transcripts out of which only three codes for the protein-androgen receptor protein.

The AR protein has three major domains, the N-terminal domain, the DNA-binding domain, and the androgen-binding domain. It belongs to a family of nuclear transcription factors. In humans, AR is present in theca interna cells and granulosa cells of preantral follicles, antral follicles, and dominant follicles. The first exon of the AR gene embeds a VNTR polymorphism consisting of CAG repeats those codes for a polyglutamine chain in the N-terminal transactivation domain.

A study by Hickey et al. reported a significantly higher frequency of alleles with longer CAG repeats (>22 repeats) in PCOS patients with infertility compared to fertile Caucasian women from Australian [87]. However, Mifsud et al. found no significant differences between the anovulatory PCOS patients and controls in the distribution of the CAG repeats [88]. Xia et al. reported that shorter alleles of the (CAG)n in the first exon of *AR* gene enhanced the PCOS susceptibility either by upregulating AR activity or resulting in hyperandrogenism in the PCOS patients from China [89] and these findings were also corroborated in the Caucasian population [90]. Rajender et al. reported that CAG bi-allelic mean length and allele distribution did not differ between controls and cases in PCOS cases from India [91].

At least two separate studies from the Chinese population have reported an association between higher serum testosterone levels in PCOS with CAG repeat length [92, 93]. Peng and coworkers reported that the SNP (rs6152G/A) leads to significantly higher susceptibility to polycystic ovary syndrome in Chinese patients [94]. Yuan et al. reported a positive correlation between GGN repeat polymorphism in the *AR* gene and PCOS in the Han Chinese population [95].

6.8 *SHBG* (sex hormone binding globulin) gene

The locus of the *SHBG* gene (ENSG00000129214) is 17p13. This gene codes for a total of 21 mRNA transcripts out of which only seventeen codes for the functional protein-sex hormone-binding globulin or sex steroid-binding globulin protein. The largest transcript (ENST00000380450.9) is 1267 bp long and has 402 amino acids with an approximate molecular weight of 90 kDa.

SHBG controls the level of sex hormones by binding to androgens, mainly with testosterone and estrogens. It is primarily synthesized by hepatocytes and controlled by multiple metabolic factors, such as androgens and insulin. The SHBG receptors are expressed in human sex-steroid-dependent cells and a wide range of tissues that include hypothalamus, colon, ovaries, prostate, etc. [96]. Concentrations of SHBG are lower in females with PCOS, due to the inhibitory effect of hyperinsulinemia on SHBG synthesis [97]. Low serum SHBG levels in PCOS women also result in hyperandrogenic symptoms such as hirsutism, acne, androgenic alopecia, and virilization [98, 99].

Hogeveen et al. reported two novel mutations, firstly, Pro156Leu, associated with abnormal glycosylation and low SHBG secretion, and a frameshift mutation in exon 8 (E326) which resulted in truncated SHBG synthesis, in a PCOS patient from France [100]. Xita et al. reported that longer allele genotypes showed a positive association with lower SHBG levels in PCOS women from Greece [101]. The same group had further reported that the combination of long *SHBG* alleles with short *CYP19* alleles results in increased testosterone levels, elevated levels of Free androgen index (FAI), Dehydroepiandrosterone-sulphate hormone (DHEAS), T/E2 ratios and low SHBG levels [102]. An independent study on PCOS women from Bahrain by Abu-Hijleh and co-workers reported that specific *SHBG* variants and haplotypes spanning six polymorphisms were linked to increased or decreased PCOS susceptibility [103].

6.9 *INS* (insulin) gene

The locus for the *INS* gene (ENSG00000254647) is 11p15.5. This gene codes for a total of 5 transcripts out of which only four codes for a functional protein. The largest transcript (ENST00000381330.5) is 465 bp long with 110 amino acids and codes for the Insulin protein. It has a variable tandem repeat (VNTR) embedded at its 5′ regulatory region ranging between 26 and 200 in number. The VNTR polymorphism in the *INS* gene has three size classes. Class-I, II and III comprises of an average length of 40, 80 and an average of 157 repeats respectively [9].

Waterworth et al. [104] reported an association of PCOS with allelic variations in the INS VNTR locus. They had observed that the class III alleles were associated with anovulatory PCOS in populations from the UK. The transmission of these allelic variations was more commonly from fathers than from mothers to affected daughters. The same study also observed that the geometric mean of fasting serum insulin concentrations was significantly higher in families with evidence of linkage [104]. Michelmore et al. demonstrated that women with polycystic ovarian morphology had increased insulin sensitivity and leptin resistance, related to insulin gene VNTR class III alleles [105].

Multiple independent studies of *INS* VNTR polymorphisms with PCOS found no signification association in Spanish [106], Czech women [107], United Kingdom, and Finland populations [108].

6.10 *INSR* (insulin receptor) gene

The locus for the *INSR* gene (ENSG00000171105) is 19p13.2. This gene has 7 available transcripts out of which only three code for the protein, insulin receptor. The largest transcript (ENST00000302850.10) is 9463 bp long with 1382 amino acids. It is a hetero-tetrameric glycoprotein composed of two α and two β-subunits and plays a significant role in insulin metabolism. The significance of the insulin signaling in PCOS is substantiated by the HAIR-AN syndrome (hyperandrogenism, insulin resistance, and acanthosis nigricans) [109]. Insulin resistance results in pituitary LH hypersecretion, increased testosterone production in theca cells, increased P450scc activity in granulosa cells, and disruption of follicular maturation, all of which contribute to PCOS susceptibility [110].

Two independent research groups have reported that the C/T SNP at His1058 in the seventeen exon of the *INSR* gene is associated with PCOS in the Caucasian and Chinese populations [111, 112]. Jin et al. reported a novel T/C polymorphism at Cys1008 resulting in decreased insulin sensitivity in Chinese PCOS women [113]. A microsatellite marker D19S884, located on chromosome 19p13.2, close to the *INSR* gene has been reported to be associated with PCOS in the Caucasian [114] and European population [115].

Mukherjee et al. found a significant association of C/T polymorphism at His1058 of the *INSR* gene in lean PCOS women while not in obese PCOS patients from Maharashtra, India [116].

6.11 *PPARG* (peroxisome proliferator-activated receptor-gamma) gene

The locus for the *PPARG* gene (ENSG00000132170) is 3p25.2. The size of the gene is approximately 100 kb with 9 exons. *PPARG* gene has a total of 34 transcripts and only twenty-two codes for the functional protein, peroxisome proliferator-activated receptor-γ. PPARG is primarily found in adipose tissue and large intestine and intermediate levels are found in the kidney, liver, and small intestine in humans and is involved in energy metabolism and adipogenesis pathway. Mutations in this gene have been linked to Partial lipodystrophy, type 2 diabetes, and dyslipidemia [117].

Hahn et al. [118] and Shaikh et al. [119] reported that a Pro12Ala polymorphism (rs1801282) of the PPARG gene in PCOS women is associated with lower hirsutism scores and increased insulin sensitivity in German and Indian population respectively. Studies by Korhonen et al. [120] and Yilmaz et al. [121] have also reported the role of this SNP in the pathogenesis of PCOS and supported its role as a protective factor against the development of diabetes mellitus in first-degree relatives of PCOS patients. Zhang et al. performed a metanalysis and reported the rs1801282 C > G polymorphism to be a protective factor in PCOS susceptibility [122].

7. Epigenetics of PCOS

The term "epigenetics" is used to describe variations that are not encoded by changes in DNA sequence and refer to several cellular elements and processes that are involved in the regulation of transcription that includes DNA modifications, non-coding RNAs, chromatin structure, and nuclear architecture. The epigenetic changes are usually transient and are heritable in daughter cells post division [123].

Wang et al. [124] reported 7929 differentially methylated CpG sites and 650 differential transcripts by combining DNA methylation profile and transcriptome analysis, in the ovaries of PCOS patients of Chinese origin. In the same study, they identified 54 genes with methylated levels correlating with gene transcription in PCOS. They also found increased hypomethylated sites and less hypermethylated sites, residing in CpG islands and N_Shore in PCOS [124]. Yu et al. [125] observed that the level of methylation was significantly higher in CpG island shores and lower within the gene bodies in Chinese cohort of PCOS patients. This study also reported that high CpG content promoters were frequently hypermethylated in PCOS ovaries but were hypomethylated in case controls [125]. Jones and coworkers identified increased methylation in the *INSR* locus and reduced methylation in the *LHCGR* locus in PCOS patients from the USA [126]. Kokosar et al. identified 440 sites with differential CpG methylation in the adipose tissue of PCOS patients [127]. Xu and coworkers [128] reported that DNA methylation altered the PCOS granulosa cells while hydroxymethylation did not have any significant effect. They identified 6936 differentially methylated CpG sites between the control and PCOS-obesity patients and 12,245 differentially methylated CpG sites were identified between the control and PCOS-nonobesity group [128]. Nillson et al. [129] found 85 differentially expressed transcripts in the skeletal muscles of PCOS patients but only two CpG sites exhibited differential DNA methylation after multiple testing. In the same study, they also reported that PCOS has epigenetic and transcriptional changes in skeletal muscle that can explain the metabolic abnormalities seen in these patients [129]. Sagvekar et al. reported that intrinsic changes in the transcriptional control of TETs and DNMT3A may contribute to DNA methylation modifications in CGCs of PCOS women in India [130].

8. Conclusion

PCOS is a serious multifactorial disorder of women in the reproductive age group resulting primarily in infertility and other gynecological issues. The etiopathology of PCOS is poorly understood. This disease presents itself differently in different ethnic groups, with few characteristics showing more in one population, and other sets of characteristics in another. While different medical organizations/associations have proposed the diagnostic criteria for PCOS based on the different clinical signs and symptoms, there is still a gray area; none of these classifications consider any molecular genetics aspects.

The role of genetic and epigenetic factors in PCOS has been widely substantiated by extensive research findings from different parts of the world in the literature. In the current book chapter, we have provided insight into the genetic and epigenetic factors that are associated with PCOS.

The results of the molecular studies along with the clinical data/ current diagnostic parameters might help in the identification of novel molecular markers to detect all PCOS phenotypes, grading the severity and in better understanding of the etiopathology of PCOS patients and thereby aiding in better clinical management.

Acknowledgements

Ms. Adity Paul acknowledges the financial support received in the form of a fellowship from Tezpur University.

Conflict of interest

The authors declare no conflict of interest.

DOI: http://dx.doi.org/10.5772/intechopen.113187

Author details

Surya Prakash Goud Ponnam* and Adity Paul
Department of Molecular Biology and Biotechnology, School of Sciences, Tezpur University, Sonitpur, Assam, India

*Address all correspondence to: surya_p@tezu.ac.in

References

[1] Stein IF, Leventhal ML. Amenorrhea associated with bilateral polycystic ovaries. American Journal of Obstetrics and Gynecology. 1935;**29**(2):181-191. DOI: 10.1016/S0002-9378(15)30642-6

[2] Sadeghi HM, Adeli I, Calina D, et al. Polycystic ovary syndrome: A comprehensive review of pathogenesis, management, and drug repurposing. International Journal of Molecular Sciences. 2022;**23**(2):583. DOI: 10.3390/ijms23020583

[3] Ding DC, Chen W, Wang JH, Lin SZ. Association between polycystic ovarian syndrome and endometrial, ovarian, and breast cancer: A population-based cohort study in Taiwan. Medicine (Baltimore). 2018;**97**(39):e12608. DOI: 10.1097/MD.0000000000012608

[4] Zehra B, Khursheed AA. Polycystic ovarian syndrome: Symptoms, treatment and diagnosis: A review. Journal of Pharmacognosy and Phytochemistry. 2018;**7**(6):875-880

[5] Jonard S, Dewailly D. The follicular excess in polycystic ovaries, due to intra-ovarian hyperandrogenism, may be the main culprit for the follicular arrest. Human Reproduction Update. 2004;**10**(2):107-117. DOI: 10.1093/humupd/dmh010

[6] Balen AH, Laven JS, Tan SL, Dewailly D. Ultrasound assessment of the polycystic ovary: International consensus definitions. Human Reproduction Update. 2003;**9**(6):505-514. DOI: 10.1093/humupd/dmg044

[7] Teede HJ, Misso ML, Costello MF, et al. Recommendations from the international evidence-based guideline for the assessment and management of polycystic ovary syndrome. Human Reproduction. 2018;**33**(9):1602-1618

[8] Moran LJ, Misso ML, Wild RA, Norman RJ. Impaired glucose tolerance, type 2 diabetes and metabolic syndrome in polycystic ovary syndrome: A systematic review and meta-analysis. Human Reproduction Update. 2010;**16**(4):347-363. DOI: 10.1093/humupd/dmq001

[9] Ataie-Ashtiani S, Forbes B. A review of the biosynthesis and structural implications of insulin gene mutations linked to human disease. Cell. 2023;**12**(7):1008. DOI: 10.3390/cells12071008

[10] Azziz R, Carmina E, Chen Z, et al. Polycystic ovary syndrome. Nature Reviews. Disease Primers. 2016;**2**:16057. DOI: 10.1038/nrdp.2016.57

[11] Liu J, Wu Q, Hao Y, et al. Measuring the global disease burden of polycystic ovary syndrome in 194 countries: Global burden of disease study 2017. Human Reproduction. 2021;**36**(4):1108-1119. DOI: 10.1093/humrep/deaa371

[12] Bulsara J, Patel P, Soni A, Acharya A. A review: Brief insight into polycystic ovarian syndrome. Endocrine and Metabolic Science. 2021;**3**:100085

[13] Ding T, Hardiman PJ, Petersen I, et al. The prevalence of polycystic ovary syndrome in reproductive-aged women of different ethnicity: A systematic review and meta-analysis. Oncotarget. 2017;**8**(56):96351-96358. DOI: 10.18632/oncotarget.19180

[14] Zhao Y, Qiao J. Ethnic differences in the phenotypic expression of polycystic ovary syndrome. Steroids.

2013;**78**(8):755-760. DOI: 10.1016/j.steroids.2013.04.006

[15] Okoroh EM, Hooper WC, Atrash HK, et al. Prevalence of polycystic ovary syndrome among the privately insured, United States, 2003-2008. American Journal of Obstetrics and Gynecology. 2012;**207**(4):299.e1-299.e7. DOI: 10.1016/j.ajog.2012.07.023

[16] Kumarapeli V, Seneviratne Rde A, Wijeyaratne CN, et al. A simple screening approach for assessing community prevalence and phenotype of polycystic ovary syndrome in a semi-urban population in Sri Lanka. American Journal of Epidemiology. 2008;**168**(3):321-328. DOI: 10.1093/aje/kwn137

[17] Tehrani FR, Simbar M, Tohidi M, et al. The prevalence of polycystic ovary syndrome in a community sample of Iranian population: Iranian PCOS prevalence study. Reproductive Biology and Endocrinology. 2011;**9**:39. DOI: 10.1186/1477-7827-9-39

[18] Yang R, Li Q, Zhou Z, et al. Changes in the prevalence of polycystic ovary syndrome in China over the past decade. Lancet Regional Health – Western Pacific. 2022;**25**:100494. DOI: 10.1016/j.lanwpc.2022.100494

[19] Gill H, Tiwari P, Dabadghao P. Prevalence of polycystic ovary syndrome in young women from North India: A community-based study. Indian Journal of Endocrinology and Metabolism. 2012;**16**(Suppl 2):S389-S392. DOI: 10.4103/2230-8210.104104

[20] Joshi B, Mukherjee S, Patil A, et al. A cross-sectional study of polycystic ovarian syndrome among adolescent and young girls in Mumbai, India. Indian Journal of Endocrinology and Metabolism. 2014;**18**(3):317-324. DOI: 10.4103/2230-8210.131162

[21] Bharali MD, Rajendran R, Goswami J, et al. Prevalence of polycystic ovarian syndrome in India: A systematic review and meta-analysis. Cureus. 2022;**14**(12):e32351. DOI: 10.7759/cureus.32351

[22] Dumesic DA, Oberfield SE, Stener-Victorin E, et al. Scientific statement on the diagnostic criteria, epidemiology, pathophysiology, and molecular genetics of polycystic ovary syndrome. Endocrine Reviews. 2015;**36**(5):487-525. DOI: 10.1210/er.2015-1018

[23] Rotterdam ESHRE/ASRM-Sponsored PCOS Consensus Workshop Group. Revised 2003 consensus on diagnostic criteria and long-term health risks related to polycystic ovary syndrome. Fertility and Sterility. 2004;**81**(1):19-25. DOI: 10.1016/j.fertnstert.2003.10.004

[24] Azziz R, Carmina E, Dewailly D, et al. The androgen excess and PCOS society criteria for the polycystic ovary syndrome: The complete task force report. Fertility and Sterility. 2009;**91**(2):456-488. DOI: 10.1016/j.fertnstert.2008.06.035

[25] Clark NM, Podolski AJ, Brooks ED, et al. Prevalence of polycystic ovary syndrome phenotypes using updated criteria for polycystic ovarian morphology: An assessment of over 100 consecutive women self-reporting features of polycystic ovary syndrome. Reproductive Sciences. 2014;**21**(8):1034-1043. DOI: 10.1177/1933719114522525

[26] Cooper HE, Spellacy WN, Prem KA, Cohen WD. Hereditary factors in the Stein-Leventhal syndrome. American Journal of Obstetrics and Gynecology.

1968;**100**(3):371-387. DOI: 10.1016/s0002-9378(15)33704-2

[27] Wilroy RS Jr, Givens JR, Wiser WL, et al. Hyperthecosis: An inheritable form of polycystic ovarian disease. Birth Defects Original Article Series. 1975;**11**(4):81-85

[28] Ferriman D, Purdie AW. The inheritance of polycystic ovarian disease and a possible relationship to premature balding. Clinical Endocrinology. 1979;**11**(3):291-300. DOI: 10.1111/j.1365-2265.1979.tb03077.x

[29] Jahanfar S, Eden JA, Warren P, et al. A twin study of polycystic ovary syndrome. Fertility and Sterility. 1995;**63**(3):478-486

[30] Vink JM, Sadrzadeh S, Lambalk CB, Boomsma DI. Heritability of polycystic ovary syndrome in a Dutch twin-family study. The Journal of Clinical Endocrinology and Metabolism. 2006;**91**(6):2100-2104. DOI: 10.1210/jc.2005-1494

[31] Heidarzadehpilehrood R, Pirhoushiaran M, Abdollahzadeh R, et al. A review on *CYP11A1*, *CYP17A1*, and *CYP19A1* polymorphism studies: Candidate susceptibility genes for polycystic ovary syndrome (PCOS) and infertility. Genes (Basel). 2022;**13**(2):302. DOI: 10.3390/genes13020302

[32] Gharani N, Waterworth DM, Batty S, et al. Association of the steroid synthesis gene CYP11a with polycystic ovary syndrome and hyperandrogenism. Human Molecular Genetics. 1997;**6**(3):397-402. DOI: 10.1093/hmg/6.3.397

[33] Diamanti-Kandarakis E, Bartzis MI, Bergiele AT, et al. Microsatellite polymorphism (tttta)(n) at −528 base pairs of gene CYP11alpha influences hyperandrogenemia in patients with polycystic ovary syndrome. Fertility and Sterility. 2000;**73**(4):735-741. DOI: 10.1016/s0015-0282(99)00628-7

[34] Wang Y, Wu XK, Cao YX, et al. Microsatellite polymorphism of (tttta) n in the promoter of CYP11a gene in Chinese women with polycystic ovary syndrome. Zhonghua Yi Xue Za Zhi. 2005;**85**(48):3396-3400

[35] Zhang CW, Zhang XL, Xia YJ, et al. Association between polymorphisms of the CYP11A1 gene and polycystic ovary syndrome in Chinese women. Molecular Biology Reports. 2012;**39**(8):8379-8385. DOI: 10.1007/s11033-012-1688-7

[36] Pusalkar M, Meherji P, Gokral J, et al. CYP11A1 and CYP17 promoter polymorphisms associate with hyperandrogenemia in polycystic ovary syndrome. Fertility and Sterility. 2009;**92**(2):653-659. DOI: 10.1016/j.fertnstert.2008.07.016

[37] Reddy KR, Deepika ML, Supriya K, et al. CYP11A1 microsatellite (tttta) n polymorphism in PCOS women from South India. Journal of Assisted Reproduction and Genetics. 2014;**31**(7):857-863. DOI: 10.1007/s10815-014-0236-x

[38] Gaasenbeek M, Powell BL, Sovio U, et al. Large-scale analysis of the relationship between CYP11A promoter variation, polycystic ovarian syndrome, and serum testosterone. The Journal of Clinical Endocrinology and Metabolism. 2004;**89**(5):2408-2413. DOI: 10.1210/jc.2003-031640

[39] Gilling-Smith C, Willis DS, Beard RW, Franks S. Hypersecretion of androstenedione by isolated thecal cells from polycystic ovaries. The Journal of Clinical Endocrinology and Metabolism.

1994;**79**(4):1158-1165. DOI: 10.1210/jcem.79.4.7962289

[40] Escobar-Morreale H, Pazos F, Potau N, et al. Ovarian suppression with triptorelin and adrenal stimulation with adrenocorticotropin in functional hyperadrogenism: Role of adrenal and ovarian cytochrome P450c17 alpha. Fertility and Sterility. 1994;**62**(3):521-530. DOI: 10.1016/s0015-0282(16)56940-4

[41] Wickenheisser JK, Nelson-DeGrave VL, Quinn PG, McAllister JM. Increased cytochrome P450 17alpha-hydroxylase promoter function in theca cells isolated from patients with polycystic ovary syndrome involves nuclear factor-1. Molecular Endocrinology. 2004;**18**(3):588-605. DOI: 10.1210/me.2003-0090

[42] Wickenheisser JK, Nelson-Degrave VL, McAllister JM. Dysregulation of cytochrome P450 17alpha-hydroxylase messenger ribonucleic acid stability in theca cells isolated from women with polycystic ovary syndrome. The Journal of Clinical Endocrinology and Metabolism. 2005;**90**(3):1720-1727. DOI: 10.1210/jc.2004-1860

[43] Carey AH, Waterworth D, Patel K, et al. Polycystic ovaries and premature male pattern baldness are associated with one allele of the steroid metabolism gene CYP17. Human Molecular Genetics. 1994;**3**(10):1873-1876. DOI: 10.1093/hmg/3.10.1873

[44] Diamanti-Kandarakis E, Bartzis MI, Zapanti ED, et al. Polymorphism T-->C (−34 bp) of gene CYP17 promoter in Greek patients with polycystic ovary syndrome. Fertility and Sterility. 1999;**71**(3):431-435. DOI: 10.1016/s0015-0282(98)00512-3

[45] Li Y, Liu F, Luo S, et al. Polymorphism T→C of gene CYP17 promoter and polycystic ovary syndrome risk: A meta-analysis. Gene. 2012;**495**(1):16-22. DOI: 10.1016/j.gene.2011.12.048

[46] Pérez MS, Cerrone GE, Benencia H, et al. Polymorphism in CYP11alpha and CYP17 genes and the etiology of hyperandrogenism in patients with polycystic ovary syndrome. Medicina (B Aires). 2008;**68**(2):129-134

[47] Kaur R, Kaur T, Kaur A. Genetic association study from North India to analyze association of CYP19A1 and CYP17A1 with polycystic ovary syndrome. Journal of Assisted Reproduction and Genetics. 2018;**35**(6):1123-1129. DOI: 10.1007/s10815-018-1162-0

[48] Gharani N, Waterworth DM, Williamson R, Franks S. 5′ polymorphism of the CYP17 gene is not associated with serum testosterone levels in women with polycystic ovaries. The Journal of Clinical Endocrinology and Metabolism. 1996;**81**(11):4174. DOI: 10.1210/jcem.81.11.8923880

[49] Marszalek B, Laciński M, Babych N, et al. Investigations on the genetic polymorphism in the region of CYP17 gene encoding 5'-UTR in patients with polycystic ovarian syndrome. Gynecological Endocrinology. 2001;**15**(2):123-128. DOI: 10.1080/gye.15.2.123.128

[50] Kahsar-Miller M, Boots LR, Bartolucci A, Azziz R. Role of a CYP17 polymorphism in the regulation of circulating dehydroepiandrosterone sulfate levels in women with polycystic ovary syndrome. Fertility and Sterility. 2004;**82**(4):973-975. DOI: 10.1016/j.fertnstert.2004.05.068

[51] Unsal T, Konac E, Yesilkaya E, et al. Genetic polymorphisms of FSHR, CYP17, CYP1A1, CAPN10, INSR, SERPINE1 genes in adolescent girls with polycystic ovary syndrome. Journal of Assisted Reproduction and Genetics. 2009;**26**(4):205-216. DOI: 10.1007/s10815-009-9308-8

[52] Simpson ER, Clyne C, Rubin G, et al. Aromatase--A brief overview. Annual Review of Physiology. 2002;**64**:93-127. DOI: 10.1146/annurev.physiol.64.081601.142703

[53] Medeiros SF, Barbosa JS, Yamamoto MM. Comparison of steroidogenic pathways among normoandrogenic and hyperandrogenic polycystic ovary syndrome patients and normal cycling women. The Journal of Obstetrics and Gynaecology Research. 2015;**41**(2):254-263. DOI: 10.1111/jog.12524

[54] Petry CJ, Ong KK, Michelmore KF, et al. Association of aromatase (CYP 19) gene variation with features of hyperandrogenism in two populations of young women. Human Reproduction. 2005;**20**(7):1837-1843. DOI: 10.1093/humrep/deh900

[55] Yu YY, Sun CX, Liu YK, et al. Promoter methylation of CYP19A1 gene in Chinese polycystic ovary syndrome patients. Gynecologic and Obstetric Investigation. 2013;**76**(4):209-213. DOI: 10.1159/000355314

[56] Chen J, Shen S, Tan Y, et al. The correlation of aromatase activity and obesity in women with or without polycystic ovary syndrome. Journal of Ovarian Research. 2015;**8**:11. DOI: 10.1186/s13048-015-0139-1

[57] Sowers MR, Wilson AL, Kardia SR, et al. Aromatase gene (CYP 19) polymorphisms and endogenous androgen concentrations in a multiracial/multiethnic, multisite study of women at midlife. The American Journal of Medicine. 2006;**119**(9 Suppl 1):S23-S30. DOI: 10.1016/j.amjmed.2006.07.003

[58] Jin JL, Sun J, Ge HJ, et al. Association between CYP19 gene SNP rs2414096 polymorphism and polycystic ovary syndrome in Chinese women. BMC Medical Genetics. 2009;**10**:139. DOI: 10.1186/1471-2350-10-139

[59] Mehdizadeh A, Kalantar SM, Sheikhha MH, et al. Association of SNP rs.2414096 CYP19 gene with polycystic ovarian syndrome in Iranian women. International Journal of Reproductive BioMedicine. 2017;**15**(8):491-496

[60] Hao CF, Zhang N, Qu Q, et al. Evaluation of the association between the CYP19 tetranucleotide (TTTA)n polymorphism and polycystic ovarian syndrome(PCOS) in Han Chinese women. Neuro Endocrinology Letters. 2010;**31**(3):370-374

[61] Lazaros L, Xita N, Hatzi E, et al. CYP19 gene variants affect the assisted reproduction outcome of women with polycystic ovary syndrome. Gynecological Endocrinology. 2013;**29**(5):478-482. DOI: 10.3109/09513590.2013.774359

[62] Ashraf S, Rasool SUA, Nabi M, et al. Impact of rs2414096 polymorphism of CYP19 gene on susceptibility of polycystic ovary syndrome and hyperandrogenism in Kashmiri women. Scientific Reports. 2021;**11**(1):12942. DOI: 10.1038/s41598-021-92265-1

[63] Dufau ML. The luteinizing hormone receptor. Annual Review of Physiology. 1998;**60**:461-496. DOI: 10.1146/annurev.physiol.60.1.461

[64] Balen AH. Hypersecretion of luteinizing hormone and the polycystic ovary syndrome. Human Reproduction. 1993;**8**(Suppl 2):123-128. DOI: 10.1093/humrep/8.suppl_2.123

[65] Furui K, Suganuma N, Tsukahara S, et al. Identification of two point mutations in the gene coding luteinizing hormone (LH) beta-subunit, associated with immunologically anomalous LH variants. The Journal of Clinical Endocrinology and Metabolism. 1994;**78**(1):107-113. DOI: 10.1210/jcem.78.1.7904610

[66] Nilsson C, Pettersson K, Millar RP, et al. Worldwide frequency of a common genetic variant of luteinizing hormone: An international collaborative research. International Collaborative Research Group. Fertility and Sterility. 1997;**67**(6):998-1004. DOI: 10.1016/s0015-0282(97)81430-6

[67] Takahashi K, Karino K, Kanasaki H, et al. Influence of missense mutation and silent mutation of LHbeta-subunit gene in Japanese patients with ovulatory disorders. European Journal of Human Genetics. 2003;**11**(5):402-408. DOI: 10.1038/sj.ejhg.5200968

[68] Chen ZJ, Zhao H, He L, et al. Genome-wide association study identifies susceptibility loci for polycystic ovary syndrome on chromosome 2p16.3, 2p21 and 9q33.3. Nature Genetics. 2011;**43**(1):55-59. DOI: 10.1038/ng.732

[69] Mutharasan P, Galdones E, Peñalver Bernabé B, et al. Evidence for chromosome 2p16.3 polycystic ovary syndrome susceptibility locus in affected women of European ancestry. The Journal of Clinical Endocrinology and Metabolism. 2013;**98**(1):E185-E190. DOI: 10.1210/jc.2012-2471

[70] Capalbo A, Sagnella F, Apa R, et al. The 312N variant of the luteinizing hormone/choriogonadotropin receptor gene (LHCGR) confers up to 2·7-fold increased risk of polycystic ovary syndrome in a Sardinian population. Clinical Endocrinology. 2012;**77**(1):113-119. DOI: 10.1111/j.1365-2265.2012.04372.x

[71] Thathapudi S, Kodati V, Erukkambattu J, et al. Association of luteinizing hormone chorionic gonadotropin receptor gene polymorphism (rs2293275) with polycystic ovarian syndrome. Genetic Testing and Molecular Biomarkers. 2015;**19**(3):128-132. DOI: 10.1089/gtmb.2014.0249

[72] Singh S, Kaur M, Kaur R, et al. Association analysis of LHCGR variants and polycystic ovary syndrome in Punjab: A case-control approach. BMC Endocrine Disorders. 2022;**22**(1):335. DOI: 10.1186/s12902-022-01251-9

[73] Urbanek M, Legro RS, Driscoll DA, et al. Thirty-seven candidate genes for polycystic ovary syndrome: Strongest evidence for linkage is with follistatin. Proceedings of the National Academy of Sciences of the United States of America. 1999;**96**(15):8573-8578. DOI: 10.1073/pnas.96.15.8573

[74] Gromoll J, Simoni M. Genetic complexity of FSH receptor function. Trends in Endocrinology and Metabolism. 2005;**16**(8):368-373. DOI: 10.1016/j.tem.2005.05.011

[75] Huhtaniemi I. The Parkes lecture. Mutations of gonadotrophin and gonadotrophin receptor genes: What do they teach us about reproductive physiology? Journal of Reproduction and Fertility. 2000;**119**(2):173-186. DOI: 10.1530/jrf.0.1190173

[76] Shi Y, Zhao H, Shi Y, et al. Genome-wide association study identifies

eight new risk loci for polycystic ovary syndrome. Nature Genetics. 2012;**44**(9):1020-1025. DOI: 10.1038/ng.2384

[77] Dolfin E, Guani B, Lussiana C, et al. FSH-receptor Ala307Thr polymorphism is associated to polycystic ovary syndrome and to a higher responsiveness to exogenous FSH in Italian women. Journal of Assisted Reproduction and Genetics. 2011;**28**(10):925-930. DOI: 10.1007/s10815-011-9619-4

[78] Gu BH, Park JM, Baek KH. Genetic variations of follicle stimulating hormone receptor are associated with polycystic ovary syndrome. International Journal of Molecular Medicine. 2010;**26**(1):107-112. DOI: 10.3892/ijmm_00000441

[79] Du J, Zhang W, Guo L, et al. Two FSHR variants, haplotypes and meta-analysis in Chinese women with premature ovarian failure and polycystic ovary syndrome. Molecular Genetics and Metabolism. 2010;**100**(3):292-295. DOI: 10.1016/j.ymgme.2010.03.018

[80] Louwers YV, Stolk L, Uitterlinden AG, Laven JS. Cross-ethnic meta-analysis of genetic variants for polycystic ovary syndrome. The Journal of Clinical Endocrinology and Metabolism. 2013;**98**(12):E2006-E2012. DOI: 10.1210/jc.2013-2495

[81] Dewailly D, Andersen CY, Balen A, et al. The physiology and clinical utility of anti-Mullerian hormone in women. Human Reproduction Update. 2014;**20**(3):370-385. DOI: 10.1093/humupd/dmt062

[82] Durlinger AL, Kramer P, Karels B, et al. Control of primordial follicle recruitment by anti-Müllerian hormone in the mouse ovary. Endocrinology. 1999;**140**(12):5789-5796. DOI: 10.1210/endo.140.12.7204

[83] Bhattacharya K, Saha I, Sen D, et al. Role of anti-Mullerian hormone in polycystic ovary syndrome. Middle East Fertility Society Journal. 2022;**27**:32. DOI: 10.1186/s43043-022-00123-5

[84] Zheng MX, Li Y, Hu R, et al. Anti-Müllerian hormone gene polymorphism is associated with androgen levels in Chinese polycystic ovary syndrome patients with insulin resistance. Journal of Assisted Reproduction and Genetics. 2016;**33**(2):199-205. DOI: 10.1007/s10815-015-0641-9

[85] Gorsic LK, Kosova G, Werstein B, et al. Pathogenic anti-Müllerian hormone variants in polycystic ovary syndrome. The Journal of Clinical Endocrinology and Metabolism. 2017;**102**(8):2862-2872. DOI: 10.1210/jc.2017-00612

[86] Kevenaar ME, Laven JS, Fong SL, et al. A functional anti-mullerian hormone gene polymorphism is associated with follicle number and androgen levels in polycystic ovary syndrome patients. The Journal of Clinical Endocrinology and Metabolism. 2008;**93**(4):1310-1316. DOI: 10.1210/jc.2007-2205

[87] Hickey T, Chandy A, Norman RJ. The androgen receptor CAG repeat polymorphism and X-chromosome inactivation in Australian Caucasian women with infertility related to polycystic ovary syndrome. The Journal of Clinical Endocrinology and Metabolism. 2002;**87**(1):161-165. DOI: 10.1210/jcem.87.1.8137

[88] Mifsud A, Ramirez S, Yong EL. Androgen receptor gene CAG trinucleotide repeats in anovulatory infertility and polycystic ovaries. The Journal of Clinical Endocrinology and Metabolism. 2000;**85**(9):3484-3488. DOI: 10.1210/jcem.85.9.6832

[89] Xia Y, Che Y, Zhang X, et al. Polymorphic CAG repeat in the androgen receptor gene in polycystic ovary syndrome patients. Molecular Medicine Reports. 2012;**5**(5):1330-1334. DOI: 10.3892/mmr.2012.789

[90] Lin LH, Baracat MC, Maciel GA, et al. Androgen receptor gene polymorphism and polycystic ovary syndrome. International Journal of Gynaecology and Obstetrics. 2013;**120**(2):115-118. DOI: 10.1016/j.ijgo.2012.08.016

[91] Rajender S, Carlus SJ, Bansal SK, et al. Androgen receptor CAG repeats length polymorphism and the risk of polycystic ovarian syndrome (PCOS). PLoS One. 2013;**8**(10):e75709. DOI: 10.1371/journal.pone.0075709

[92] Kim JJ, Choung SH, Choi YM, et al. Androgen receptor gene CAG repeat polymorphism in women with polycystic ovary syndrome. Fertility and Sterility. 2008;**90**(6):2318-2323. DOI: 10.1016/j.fertnstert.2007.10.030

[93] Peng CY, Xie HJ, Guo ZF, et al. The association between androgen receptor gene CAG polymorphism and polycystic ovary syndrome: A case-control study and meta-analysis. Journal of Assisted Reproduction and Genetics. 2014;**31**(9):1211-1219. DOI: 10.1007/s10815-014-0286-0

[94] Peng CY, Long XY, Lu GX. Association of AR rs6152G/a gene polymorphism with susceptibility to polycystic ovary syndrome in Chinese women. Reproduction, Fertility, and Development. 2010;**22**(5):881-885. DOI: 10.1071/RD09190

[95] Yuan C, Gao C, Qian Y, et al. Polymorphism of CAG and GGN repeats of androgen receptor gene in women with polycystic ovary syndrome. Reproductive Biomedicine Online. 2015;**31**(6):790-798. DOI: 10.1016/j.rbmo.2015.09.007

[96] Rosner W, Hryb DJ, Kahn SM, et al. Interactions of sex hormone-binding globulin with target cells. Molecular and Cellular Endocrinology. 2010;**316**(1):79-85. DOI: 10.1016/j.mce.2009.08.009

[97] Nestler JE, Powers LP, Matt DW, et al. A direct effect of hyperinsulinemia on serum sex hormone-binding globulin levels in obese women with the polycystic ovary syndrome. The Journal of Clinical Endocrinology and Metabolism. 1991;**72**(1):83-89. DOI: 10.1210/jcem-72-1-83

[98] Rannevik G, Jeppsson S, Johnell O, et al. A longitudinal study of the perimenopausal transition: Altered profiles of steroid and pituitary hormones, SHBG and bone mineral density. Maturitas. 1995;**21**(2):103-113. DOI: 10.1016/0378-5122(94)00869-9

[99] Burger HG, Dudley EC, Cui J, et al. A prospective longitudinal study of serum testosterone, dehydroepiandrosterone sulfate, and sex hormone-binding globulin levels through the menopause transition. The Journal of Clinical Endocrinology and Metabolism. 2000;**85**(8):2832-2838. DOI: 10.1210/jcem.85.8.6740

[100] Hogeveen KN, Cousin P, Pugeat M, et al. Human sex hormone-binding globulin variants associated with hyperandrogenism and ovarian dysfunction. The Journal of Clinical Investigation. 2002;**109**(7):973-981. DOI: 10.1172/JCI14060

[101] Xita N, Tsatsoulis A, ChatzikyriakidouA,GeorgiouI.Association of the (TAAAA)n repeat polymorphism in the sex hormone-binding globulin (SHBG) gene with polycystic ovary

syndrome and relation to SHBG serum levels. The Journal of Clinical Endocrinology and Metabolism. 2003;**88**(12):5976-5980. DOI: 10.1210/jc.2003-030197

[102] Xita N, Georgiou I, Lazaros L, et al. The synergistic effect of sex hormone-binding globulin and aromatase genes on polycystic ovary syndrome phenotype. European Journal of Endocrinology. 2008;**158**(6):861-865. DOI: 10.1530/EJE-07-0905

[103] Abu-Hijleh TM, Gammoh E, Al-Busaidi AS, et al. Common variants in the sex hormone-binding globulin (SHBG) gene influence SHBG levels in women with polycystic ovary syndrome. Annals of Nutrition & Metabolism. 2016;**68**(1):66-74. DOI: 10.1159/000441570

[104] Waterworth DM, Bennett ST, Gharani N, et al. Linkage and association of insulin gene VNTR regulatory polymorphism with polycystic ovary syndrome. Lancet. 1997;**349**(9057):986-990. DOI: 10.1016/S0140-6736(96)08368-7

[105] Michelmore K, Ong K, Mason S, et al. Clinical features in women with polycystic ovaries: Relationships to insulin sensitivity, insulin gene VNTR and birth weight. Clinical Endocrinology. 2001;**55**(4):439-446. DOI: 10.1046/j.1365-2265.2001.01375.x

[106] Calvo RM, Tellería D, Sancho J, et al. Insulin gene variable number of tandem repeats regulatory polymorphism is not associated with hyperandrogenism in Spanish women. Fertility and Sterility. 2002;**77**(4):666-668. DOI: 10.1016/s0015-0282(01)03238-1

[107] Vanková M, Vrbíková J, Hill M, et al. Association of insulin gene VNTR polymorphism with polycystic ovary syndrome. Annals of the New York Academy of Sciences. 2002;**967**:558-565. DOI: 10.1111/j.1749-6632.2002.tb04317.x

[108] Powell BL, Haddad L, Bennett A, et al. Analysis of multiple data sets reveals no association between the insulin gene variable number tandem repeat element and polycystic ovary syndrome or related traits. The Journal of Clinical Endocrinology and Metabolism. 2005;**90**(5):2988-2993. DOI: 10.1210/jc.2004-2485

[109] Rager KM, Omar HA. Androgen excess disorders in women: The severe insulin-resistant hyperandrogenic syndrome, HAIR-AN. Scientific World Journal. 2006;**6**:116-121. DOI: 10.1100/tsw.2006.23

[110] Diamanti-Kandarakis E, Papavassiliou AG. Molecular mechanisms of insulin resistance in polycystic ovary syndrome. Trends in Molecular Medicine. 2006;**12**(7):324-332. DOI: 10.1016/j.molmed.2006.05.006

[111] Siegel S, Futterweit W, Davies TF, et al. A C/T single nucleotide polymorphism at the tyrosine kinase domain of the insulin receptor gene is associated with polycystic ovary syndrome. Fertility and Sterility. 2002;**78**(6):1240-1243. DOI: 10.1016/s0015-0282(02)04241-3

[112] Chen ZJ, Shi YH, Zhao YR, et al. Correlation between single nucleotide polymorphism of insulin receptor gene with polycystic ovary syndrome. Zhonghua Fu Chan Ke Za Zhi. 2004;**39**(9):582-585

[113] Jin L, Zhu XM, Luo Q, et al. A novel SNP at exon 17 of INSR is associated with decreased insulin sensitivity in Chinese women with PCOS. Molecular Human Reproduction. 2006;**12**(3):151-155. DOI: 10.1093/molehr/gal022

[114] Tucci S, Futterweit W, Concepcion ES, et al. Evidence for association of polycystic ovary syndrome in caucasian women with a marker at the insulin receptor gene locus. The Journal of Clinical Endocrinology and Metabolism. 2001;**86**(1):446-449. DOI: 10.1210/jcem.86.1.7274

[115] Urbanek M, Woodroffe A, Ewens KG, et al. Candidate gene region for polycystic ovary syndrome on chromosome 19p13.2. The Journal of Clinical Endocrinology and Metabolism. 2005;**90**(12):6623-6629. DOI: 10.1210/jc.2005-0622

[116] Mukherjee S, Shaikh N, Khavale S, et al. Genetic variation in exon 17 of INSR is associated with insulin resistance and hyperandrogenemia among lean Indian women with polycystic ovary syndrome. European Journal of Endocrinology. 2009;**160**(5):855-862. DOI: 10.1530/EJE-08-0932

[117] Janani C, Ranjitha Kumari BD. PPAR gamma gene--a review. Diabetes and Metabolic Syndrome: Clinical Research and Reviews. 2015;**9**(1):46-50. DOI: 10.1016/j.dsx.2014.09.015

[118] Hahn S, Fingerhut A, Khomtsiv U, et al. The peroxisome proliferator activated receptor gamma Pro12Ala polymorphism is associated with a lower hirsutism score and increased insulin sensitivity in women with polycystic ovary syndrome. Clinical Endocrinology. 2005;**62**(5):573-579. DOI: 10.1111/j.1365-2265.2005.02261

[119] Shaikh N, Mukherjee A, Shah N, et al. Peroxisome proliferator activated receptor gamma gene variants influence susceptibility and insulin related traits in Indian women with polycystic ovary syndrome. Journal of Assisted Reproduction and Genetics. 2013;**30**(7):913-921. DOI: 10.1007/s10815-013-0025-y

[120] Korhonen S, Heinonen S, Hiltunen M, et al. Polymorphism in the peroxisome proliferator-activated receptor-gamma gene in women with polycystic ovary syndrome. Human Reproduction. 2003;**18**(3):540-543. DOI: 10.1093/humrep/deg128

[121] Yilmaz M, Ergün MA, Karakoç A, et al. Pro12Ala polymorphism of the peroxisome proliferator-activated receptor-gamma gene in first-degree relatives of subjects with polycystic ovary syndrome. Gynecological Endocrinology. 2005;**21**(4):206-210. DOI: 10.1080/09513590500231593

[122] Zhang S, Wang Y, Jiang H, et al. Peroxisome proliferator-activated receptor gamma rs1801282 C>G polymorphism is associated with polycystic ovary syndrome susceptibility: A meta-analysis involving 7,069 subjects. International Journal of Clinical and Experimental Medicine. 2015;**8**(10):17418-17429

[123] Stener-Victorin E, Deng Q. Epigenetic inheritance of polycystic ovary syndrome — Challenges and opportunities for treatment. Nature Reviews. Endocrinology. 2021;**17**:521-533. DOI: 10.1038/s41574-021-00517

[124] Wang XX, Wei JZ, Jiao J, et al. Genome-wide DNA methylation and gene expression patterns provide insight into polycystic ovary syndrome development. Oncotarget. 2014;**5**(16):6603-6610. DOI: 10.18632/oncotarget.2224

[125] Yu YY, Sun CX, Liu YK, et al. Genome-wide screen of ovary-specific DNA methylation in polycystic ovary syndrome. Fertility and Sterility. 2015;**104**(1):145-53.e6. DOI: 10.1016/j.fertnstert.2015.04.005

[126] Jones MR, Brower MA, Xu N, et al. Systems genetics reveals the functional

context of PCOS loci and identifies genetic and molecular mechanisms of disease heterogeneity. PLoS Genetics. 2015;**11**(8):e1005455. DOI: 10.1371/journal.pgen.1005455

[127] Kokosar M, Benrick A, Perfilyev A, et al. Epigenetic and transcriptional alterations in human adipose tissue of polycystic ovary syndrome. Scientific Reports. 2016;**6**:22883. DOI: 10.1038/srep22883

[128] Xu J, Bao X, Peng Z, et al. Comprehensive analysis of genome-wide DNA methylation across human polycystic ovary syndrome ovary granulosa cell. Oncotarget. 2016;**7**(19):27899-27909. DOI: 10.18632/oncotarget.8544

[129] Nilsson E, Benrick A, Kokosar M, et al. Transcriptional and epigenetic changes influencing skeletal muscle metabolism in women with polycystic ovary syndrome. The Journal of Clinical Endocrinology and Metabolism. 2018;**103**(12):4465-4477. DOI: 10.1210/jc.2018-00935

[130] Sagvekar P, Shinde G, Mangoli V, et al. Evidence for TET-mediated DNA demethylation as an epigenetic alteration in cumulus granulosa cells of women with polycystic ovary syndrome. Molecular Human Reproduction. 2022;**28**(7):gaac019. DOI: 10.1093/molehr/gaac019

Chapter 2

Optimizing Nutrition for PCOS Management: A Comprehensive Guide

Madan Pandey and Kritee Niroula

Abstract

This chapter aims to provide a comprehensive guide to optimizing nutrition for the management of polycystic ovary syndrome (PCOS), a hormonal disorder affecting reproductive-aged women that are associated with various metabolic and reproductive complications. It explores the critical role of nutrition in PCOS management, focusing on evidence-based dietary strategies to alleviate symptoms, promote hormonal balance, and enhance overall health outcomes. Beginning with the pathophysiology of PCOS, the chapter highlights the impact of insulin resistance, inflammation, and hormonal imbalances on the condition. The chapter provides practical guidelines for optimizing macronutrient intake, including recommendations for carbohydrate quality, protein sources, and fat composition. Additionally, it explores the potential benefits of dietary supplements and herbal remedies in PCOS management. It addresses key lifestyle factors—physical activity, stress management, and adequate sleep—which synergistically enhance nutrition in optimizing PCOS management. This valuable resource is tailored for healthcare professionals, nutritionists, and individuals with PCOS seeking evidence-based guidance on effectively managing this complex condition through optimized nutrition.

Keywords: polycystic ovary syndrome, endocrine-metabolic disorder, nutrition in PCOS, dietary therapy, dietary supplements

1. Introduction

Polycystic ovary syndrome (PCOS) is an endocrine-metabolic disorder affecting women of reproductive age [1]. It is a heterogeneous endocrine condition characterized by elevated androgen levels and endocrine variation, menstrual irregularities, and anovulation and/or small cysts on one or both ovaries that severely impact the life of a woman [2–4]. PCOS, marked by enlarged ovaries and amenorrhea, was characterized in 1935 by Stein and Leventhal. Extensive research since then aims to understand its molecular mechanisms and improve management. PCOS involves a complex interplay of genetic and environmental factors [5]. PCOS, known for reproductive issues, also poses metabolic risks like obesity, diabetes, and cardiovascular diseases. It adversely affects mental health, reducing quality of life. Weight reduction through lifestyle changes is crucial for managing and improving the reproductive, metabolic, and psychological aspects of PCOS. Thus, lifestyle changes should be the primary management approach for PCOS [6].

2. Polycystic ovarian (PCO) physiology

The ovarian follicles are functional units of the mammalian ovary, which are roughly spheroid cellular aggregations consisting of an oocyte (germ cell) surrounded by granulosa cells forming intercellular connections and further surrounded by theca cells [7, 8]. There are approximately 295,000 primordial follicles in the ovarian reserve per ovary of a female human child at birth [9, 10]. Follicular growth is coordinated, usually resulting in the selection of a single follicle for maturation and ovulation sequentially. Over time, the continual recruitment of more primordial follicles from this pool is a dynamic process. The regulation of the rate at which primordial follicles enter the growing pool has a crucial role in maintaining the ovarian reserve and safeguarding fertility. However, during PCOS, due to a potential dysregulation in the recruitment mechanism of primordial follicles for growth, a greater number of small antral follicles (2–9 mm in diameter) are formed than in the normal ovary. During a normal menstrual cycle, the luteinizing hormone (LH) response is limited to the dominant follicle, usually when it attains a diameter of around 10 mm. However, in individuals with PCOS, the LH response occurs unusually in smaller follicles. Consequently, a significant proportion of antral follicles undergo terminal differentiation before the appropriate time. As the antral follicles produce steroids (estrogen) and inhibin B, the presence of a large number of these follicles results in an increased production of a higher amount of steroids (estrogen) and inhibin B. They have negative feedback on the production of follicle-stimulating hormone (FSH). As FSH has a role in the maturation of the follicles and the release of the ovum, its imbalance leads to the arrest of follicular growth and the ovum is not released, creating a large number of cysts-like structures containing immature ovum [11–13]. PCOS is distinguished by an elevated count of follicles across all developmental stages, with a notable increase observed in the pre-antral and small antral follicles [14].

3. Pathophysiology of PCOS

PCOS is a complex endocrine disorder involving genetics, environment, obesity, ovarian dysfunction, and hormonal imbalances like elevated androgens and hyperinsulinemia. It disrupts the hypothalamic-pituitary-ovarian (HPO) axis and leads to symptoms of excess androgens and irregular ovulation [6, 15]. Hyperandrogenism, often characterized by elevated levels of unbound (free) testosterone in the blood, is the prevailing anomaly in this syndrome and plays a significant role in perpetuating the irregular hormonal factors contributing to the pathophysiology of PCOS. PCOS is complex, with disruptions in the menstrual cycle, hyperandrogenism, and obesity. Ovarian dysfunction is crucial to its pathophysiology, involving multiple factors and genes [16]. Here are some of the complications of PCOS:

3.1 Hyperandrogenism

Clinical and biochemical hyperandrogenism are major features of PCOS. Disruptions in hypothalamic-pituitary feedback, excessive LH secretion, premature

DOI: http://dx.doi.org/10.5772/intechopen.114149

luteinization of granulosa cells, irregular oocyte maturation, and premature arrest of activated primary follicles are associated with persistent hyperandrogenism [15]. Excessive ovarian androgen production is the result of a combination of intrinsic ovarian factors, such as alterations in steroidogenesis, and external factors, such as hyperinsulinemia [15].

3.2 Polycystic ovaries, ovulatory dysfunction

A well-coordinated interaction of reproductive, metabolic, and intraovarian processes is necessary for ovulation. Follicle development is disrupted by ovarian hyperandrogenism, hyperinsulinemia due to insulin resistance (IR), and altered intraovarian paracrine signaling during PCOS. This disruption leads to follicular arrest, resulting in menstrual irregularities, anovulatory subfertility, and the accumulation of small antral follicles in the ovarian periphery, which imparts a polycystic morphology to the ovary [17].

3.3 Insulin resistance (IR), impaired lipid metabolism, obesity

Excessive levels of androgens influence where fat is stored in the body. The pattern of fat accumulation is altered in hyperandrogenic women with PCOS [18]. Testosterone promotes visceral fat accumulation and IR [19]. Hyperinsulinemia then further exacerbates androgen generation. The anabolic effect of hyperinsulinemia on fat metabolism via the adipogenesis process results in an elevated uptake of glucose into adipocytes and the subsequent production of triglycerides, contributing to obesity [20]. Central obesity is a distinctive feature of PCOS, as evidenced by an elevated waist-to-hip ratio in these patients compared to obese women without PCOS. Hyperinsulinemia may contribute to the development of central adiposity, further exacerbating underlying or latent IR [21].

4. Complications and symptoms

4.1 Menstrual abnormalities

Chronic anovulation often manifests as various forms of menstrual irregularities such as secondary amenorrhea, oligomenorrhea, and dysfunctional uterine bleeding [21]. In PCOS, irregular menstrual cycles begin at menarche or shortly after, often progressing to oligomenorrhea or amenorrhea. Menstrual dysfunction, marked by anovulation and unpredictable bleeding, correlates with IR severity. Longer cycles, beyond 3 months, indicate higher IR. Amenorrhea in PCOS exacerbates IR. Prolonged anovulation results in irregular bleeding resembling regular periods. Chronic anovulation, especially in obesity, leads to atypical endometrial thickening, a precursor to endometrial cancer [20].

4.2 Hirsutism, acne, and male pattern alopecia

Hirsutism, acne, and male pattern alopecia are manifestations of hyperandrogenism. Hirsutism, the growth of coarse pigmented hairs in androgen-dependent areas, including the face, chest, back, and lower abdomen, is driven by testosterone and dihydrotestosterone [20, 21].

Androgenic alopecia, a form of hair loss, is a less well-studied marker for androgen excess [16]. The balding pattern primarily affects the frontal and parietal scalp zones, with the occipital area maintaining a higher hair density [20].

In PCOS, acne is exacerbated because sebaceous glands, influenced by androgens, are sensitive structures that contribute to acne and seborrhoea intensified by sebaceous gland sensitivity [16, 20]. Androgens stimulate the proliferation of sebocytes and the secretion of sebum, which comprises lipids such as glycerides, squalene, free fatty acids (FFA), and cholesterol.

4.3 Dyslipidaemia

The majority of PCOS patients exhibit dyslipidaemia, driven by factors like insulin, estrogen, and androgens influencing lipoprotein lipid metabolism. Elevated hepatic lipase activity, stimulated by insulin, plays a role in lipid alterations. Hyperandrogenism is linked to adverse lipid profiles, particularly testosterone's negative impact on lipids. The typical lipid profile in PCOS features elevated low-density lipoprotein (LDL) cholesterol, increased very low-density lipoprotein (VLDL) cholesterol, higher triglycerides, and reduced high-density lipoprotein (HDL) cholesterol. These lipid issues worsen in PCOS women with glucose intolerance [20].

4.4 Non-alcoholic fatty liver disease (NFALD)

Common pathophysiological factors linking NAFLD and PCOS include obesity and IR. Elevated liver enzymes and IR are associated with both conditions. NAFLD worsens IR, aggravating it in PCOS. Conversely, IR leads to lipolysis, increasing hepatic fat accumulation and collagen production. Hyperandrogenism is linked to IR and affects NAFLD independently of it. Hyperandrogenic women with PCOS tend to have a higher liver fat [22].

4.5 Chronic inflammation, endothelial function, and atherosclerosis

Chronic inflammation, endothelial dysfunction, and atherosclerosis are key considerations in understanding cardiovascular implications of PCOS. Endothelial injury is an early indication of cardiovascular issues. Testosterone levels in hyperandrogenic insulin-resistant women correlate with abnormal endothelial function. Mechanisms include reduced nitric oxide synthesis, enhanced inactivation, increased vasoconstrictor synthesis, and insulin's direct effects. Obesity exacerbates endothelial dysfunction and reduced adiponectin in PCOS further contributes. PCOS, a proinflammatory state, links chronic inflammation to metabolic and ovarian dysfunction. Elevated C-reactive protein promotes atherosclerosis and endothelial cell inflammation, raising cardiovascular risk [20].

4.6 Gestational diabetes mellitus (GDM) and diabetes mellitus (DM)

In a typical pregnancy, maternal carbohydrate metabolism changes, including pancreatic β-cell hyperplasia and increased insulin sensitivity, followed by the development of insulin resistance (IR). Women with PCOS, already predisposed to IR, face a higher risk of gestational diabetes mellitus (GDM) due to these changes. The pathophysiology involves IR and abnormalities in β-cell glucose sensitivity, resulting in inadequate insulin response. Pregnancy-related IR, combined with pre-existing IR in

PCOS, heightens the risk. PCOS women with GDM also face an increased likelihood of impaired glucose tolerance post-delivery. Their heightened risk of progressing to impaired glucose metabolism and type II diabetes (T2D) is influenced by a prevalent family history of T2D. Diabetes may contribute more significantly to mortality rates in PCOS women compared to the general population [20].

4.7 Infertility and recurrent pregnancy loss (RPL)

PCOS often leads to anovulatory infertility, but some women with PCOS can conceive, though with longer conception times. In cases of infertility, overweight is common among PCOS-affected women. RPL occurs in PCOS, with uncertain reasons like uterine dysfunction, disrupted cell-embryo interaction, or insulin-related factors. PCOS mainly affects fertility through oligo-ovulation or anovulation. High LH concentrations during the follicular phase can reduce conception rates and cause early pregnancy loss. LH hypersecretion in PCOS may trigger premature oocyte maturation and impact folliculogenesis, leading to endometrial receptivity issues. Hyperinsulinemia in PCOS might hinder preimplantation conditions and affect embryo-endometrial interaction, contributing to pregnancy loss [20, 21].

5. Etiology, causes and associated factors

PCOS is a complex polygenic disorder resulting from the interplay of various genetic, environmental, and intrauterine influences, with an estimated heritability of about 70% [13, 23]. Several susceptible genes have been identified as contributors to the pathophysiology of the. Additionally, the environment plays a major role in the expression of these genes and the development and progression of the disease. The most common environmental factors include obesity and IR [24–27]. Some factors that can lead to PCOS are:

5.1 Heredity and genetic linkages

PCOS often runs in families, showing a dominant trait inheritance pattern. Twin studies highlight family factors in PCOS. Maternal PCOS, PCOM (polycystic ovarian morphology), hyperandrogenaemia, and metabolic syndrome are heritable risk factors. Daughters of PCOS women exhibit elevated AMH in infancy, larger ovaries, and increased insulin responses in childhood. Post-menarche, they may have higher testosterone. PCOM tends to follow an inherited pattern, with sisters having a higher risk of PCOM, hirsutism, and irregular periods. Parental factors and defective insulin secretion contribute, leading to increased adiposity, abnormal glucose tolerance, and diabetes in relatives. Gene variants are associated with PCOS [28].

5.2 Intrauterine environment

There is growing evidence that developmental exposure to a distorted environment can induce enduring alterations in the epigenome. These modifications subsequently contribute to altered gene expression and an elevated susceptibility to adult-onset diseases. Factors such as congenital virilization and intrauterine nutrition have been recognized as potential contributors to the risk of developing PCOS [28].

5.3 Postnatal environment

Postnatal environmental factors can trigger latent, congenitally programmed susceptibility traits to surface as PCOS symptoms. Key factors include:

Insulin resistance: PCOS is linked to extreme IR, with high insulin levels contributing to anovulation. Weight loss and improved insulin sensitivity enhance ovulation and menstrual cyclicity [28].

Hyperandrogenism: postnatal androgen excess, observed in some animal models and conditions like congenital adrenal virilizing disorders, contributes to ovarian hyperandrogenism [28].

Obesity: obesity, independently and by exacerbating PCOS, increases reproductive features—hyperandrogenism, hirsutism, infertility and pregnancy complications. Additionally, obesity amplifies the risk factors associated with PCOS, such as impaired glucose tolerance, T2D, and cardiovascular disease (CVD) [29].

6. Nutrition in PCOS

Some evolutionary biologists posit that numerous genetic and hormonal predispositions contributing to PCOS may have originated during the transition from a pre-agrarian age diet to a contemporary diet. This hypothesis is substantiated by the concurrent increase in rates of diabetes, heart disease, and PCOS, aligning with the swift changes in the modern human diet. For all women diagnosed with PCOS, the inclusion of dietary therapy and regular exercise offers noteworthy benefits. Indeed, dietary and lifestyle interventions are regarded as primary strategies for managing PCOS. While there is not a specific "PCOS diet" that can completely reverse the syndrome, several dietary principles should be followed to ameliorate its symptoms [30].

A growing body of evidence indicates that various dietary strategies might yield positive effects on PCOS features, even without resulting in weight loss. Here, the impact of different nutrients and other dietary modifications according to diet strategies will be discussed.

6.1 Different nutrients in PCOS

6.1.1 Dietary carbohydrates

There is no optimum amount of carbohydrate intake for women with PCOS, and, therefore, any range (about 40–55%) of dietary carbohydrates can be adopted, according to the individuals' dietary assessment, metabolic goals, dietary habits and preferences. However, a beneficial strategy might involve consuming a larger portion of carbohydrates during lunchtime. Another appropriate approach would be to evenly spread carbohydrates across meals throughout the day. It would be better to avoid having a high-carbohydrate breakfast. While limited, studies have been done incorporating low-glycaemic index (GI) foods that might offer slight additional benefits for certain PCOS outcomes [31].

6.1.2 Protein

Studies have found a diet higher in protein may yield several positive health outcomes, including increased weight loss, preservation of lean mass during weight loss and maintenance, improved glycaemic control, and mitigation of other CVD risk factors such as blood pressure. However, it remains unclear whether these effects are primarily attributable to the higher protein intake or a reduction in carbohydrate intake. Some factors like increased thermogenesis and enhanced satiety have been proposed. Adding 7–15 g of dietary protein to meals and snacks might offer health benefits for women with PCOS, particularly regarding insulin sensitivity and post-prandial glucose levels [31].

6.1.3 Fat

It has been found that low-fat hypocaloric diets can help reduce body weight and composition compared to high-fat hypocaloric diets. Moderately low-carbohydrate, high-fat diets can help to decrease fasting insulin, increase insulin sensitivity, and improve metabolic parameters in women with PCOS. Furthermore, a diet moderately low in carbohydrates (43%) but rich in unsaturated fatty acids may lead to a significant decline in fasting insulin levels A diet rich in fat and moderately limited in carbohydrates (~41% carbohydrate, 19% protein, 40% fat) may significantly reduce in basal β-cell response, fasting insulin, fasting glucose, and IR and decrease testosterone levels, in conjunction with declines in blood lipid levels and adipose tissue mass [31].

6.1.4 Micronutrients

Women with PCOS often have imbalanced diets with deficiencies in essential nutrients such as fiber, Ω-3 fatty acids, calcium, magnesium, zinc, and vitamins (folic acid, vitamin C, vitamin B12, and vitamin D). There is also an excess intake of certain nutrients like sucrose, sodium, total fats, saturated fatty acids, and cholesterol. Balancing deficiencies with a calorie-reduced diet with a low GI can positively influence water-soluble vitamins [32]. While most B vitamins respond well to increased dietary supply, a study has shown that such an effect may not be observed for vitamins B_3, B_2 and thiamine [33]. Women with PCOS are treated with metformin, but its chronic intake may lead to deficiencies in thiamine and cobalamin [34]. So, these vitamin supplementations may be necessary.

Micronutrients like selenium, chromium, zinc, carotenoids, and vitamin E can have potential benefits in the metabolic condition of PCOS patients and deficiency in these nutrients might contribute to the exacerbation of metabolic disturbances in PCOS patients with metabolic syndromes [35]. Supplementation of micronutrients like zinc, selenium, chromium, and folate may positively impact fasting glucose, insulin, IR, blood lipid levels, and inflammatory and oxidative stress biomarkers in PCOS individuals. Despite potential benefits, recommending micronutrient supplements for PCOS management is considered premature based on current evidence [31, 36]. Thus, the consumption of micronutrient-rich foods on a daily basis becomes important.

6.2 Dietary strategies

6.2.1 Negative energy balance and weight reduction

Calorie restriction diets (1000–1500 kcal/day) can help in weight loss and improvements in hirsutism, IR, and androgen levels [37]. Modest weight loss (5–10%) in PCOS shows positive impacts on cardiovascular and diabetes risk, hormone levels, and PCOS outcomes. Weight reduction yields improved insulin sensitivity and lipid profiles, alleviating hyperandrogenism, increased Sex hormone Binding Globulin (SHBG), reduced Free Androgen Index (FAI) and testosterone, and normalizing menstrual cycles. Weight loss benefits overweight PCOS women by reducing IR and hyperandrogenism and enhancing ovarian health, menstrual function, and ovulation. Effects on LH vary, while hirsutism may improve. The extent of the caloric deficit should be tailored to individual needs, including dietary preferences, habits, cultural factors, metabolic objectives, and physical activity levels [31].

6.2.2 Glycaemic index and glycaemic load

From different studies, it has been found that low-GI diets are helpful for successful weight loss, increase insulin sensitivity, and reduce IR, fasting insulin, LDL cholesterol, triglycerides, waist circumference, total testosterone and maintaining menstrual regularity when compared to high GI diets. A low to medium glycaemic load (GL) diet containing high-protein, moderately low-carb can also be helpful for improvement in IR, and inflammation markers. Low-GI foods, however, have similar effects as conventional diets on fasting glucose, HDL cholesterol, free androgen, inflammation, and quality of life [31, 32].

6.2.3 Meal frequency

Meal frequency and timing are important considerations in lifestyle changes for PCOS management, although there is limited specific data for women with PCOS. There are contrasting viewpoints on the effects of meal frequency on body composition and glycaemic control. Some argue that frequent meals might lead to weight gain due to increased fat deposition after meals or higher energy intake. Others suggest that increased meal frequency could spread nutrient load, leading to lower postprandial insulin levels, reduced hunger, and improved glucose clearance. In a study, a six-meal pattern showed improved post-oral glucose tolerance test insulin sensitivity and reduced subjective hunger in women with PCOS compared to a three-meal pattern. Another study showed that consuming a high-energy breakfast instead of a high-energy dinner improved insulin sensitivity and reproductive markers in lean women with PCOS. Meal timing has also gained attention. Eating late in the day has been linked to decreased energy expenditure, impaired glucose tolerance, and disrupted circadian rhythms. People with prediabetes who prefer evening meals might have a higher risk of developing T2D. The American Heart Association suggests that meal frequency and timing could be crucial in managing chronic diseases and reducing cardiometabolic risk factors [31].

6.2.4 Dietary modification

Multiple dietary compositions show promise in treating obesity and its associated conditions in PCOS [29]. Implementing low-GI diets, exercise, and omega-3 supplementation leads to increased HDL, SHBG synthesis, and reduced body fat. Studies support the efficacy and safety of the low-GI diet in relieving IR, and proper professional dietary advice should be provided for PCOS patients [32].

The DASH diet, which is low-GI and high in complex carbohydrates, demonstrated positive effects on weight loss, insulin metabolism, and inflammation markers in women with PCOS. Adherence to the DASH diet led to significant reductions in body weight, insulin levels, IR, high-sensitivity C-reactive protein, and triglycerides, encouraging healthy dietary patterns like DASH or Mediterranean-style diets, rich in fiber, antioxidants, and anti-inflammatory nutrients, could be beneficial for women with PCOS due to their satiety, anti-hyperlipidaemic, antihypertensive, and anti-diabetic properties [31].

Low-carbohydrate diets (<30% of energy) contribute to weight loss and metabolic enhancements. Specifically, long-term low-carb diets, including low-fat/low-carb variations, are recommended to reduce BMI, address PCOS with IR, prevent high LDL-C, increase FSH and SHBG levels, and decrease total testosterone. Controlled carbohydrate intake positively affects PCOS aspects, presenting a significant intervention for symptom improvement [37, 38]. Studies suggest that a high-protein, low-carb diet may aid weight loss and improve metabolic and reproductive parameters in PCOS. Carbohydrate restriction, especially with a low glycaemic index (GI), is proposed for satiety and cardiovascular health, though sustaining long-term adherence proves challenging (**Table 1**) [29].

6.3 Dietary supplements in PCOS management

6.3.1 Omega-3 fatty acids

Omega-3 fatty acids, often lacking in PCOS diets, enhance reproductive performance by affecting hormone secretion and ovarian functions [32]. Omega-3 fatty acids, specifically EPA and DHA, offer various positive effects, such as antioxidant, anti-inflammatory, anti-obesity, and insulin-sensitizing properties. They enhance insulin sensitivity by reducing inflammatory cytokines and boosting anti-inflammatory adiponectin secretion in PCOS women, which is evident through decreased

1. Adjust according to standard levels for sex, age, and activity. Implement a 500–1000 kcal/day reduction for effective weight loss (7–10% over 6–12 months).
2. For nutritionally complete dietary patterns include:
    - Low-fat dairy (two to three servings/day)
    - Whole-grain/low-GI bread and cereals (at least three servings/day)
    - Fruit (at least two servings/day)
    - Vegetables (at least two cups/day)
    - Lean meat, chicken, fish (one to two serves/day)
    - Low-saturated fat fats/oils (three to four teaspoons or nuts/seeds)
3. Maintain <10% of calories from saturated fat.
4. Increase consumption of fiber, whole-grain bread, cereals, and fruits/vegetables.
5. Increasing dietary protein or unrefined carbohydrates equally improves reproductive and metabolic parameters.
6. Reduce refined carbohydrates, favoring complex carbohydrates.
7. Include low glycaemic index foods in the diet.
8. Increase fiber Intake to enhance glucose regulation.
9. Emphasize high-protein foods, particularly at breakfast, for greater fullness, increased satiety, and reduced ghrelin concentrations.
10. Maintain a regular eating pattern for optimal results.

Table 1.
Dietary recommendations for PCOS [39].

high-sensitivity C-reactive protein and increased adiponectin levels. However, the impact of omega-3 supplementation on PCOS remains debated, with mixed study results on waist circumference, lipid profiles, and menstrual regularity. Studies indicate that n-3 PUFA supplementation may reduce total testosterone levels, while further research is required to explore the potential antiandrogenic effects of long-chain n-3 PUFAs, including EPA and DHA [31].

6.3.2 Vitamin D

The complex interplay between vitamin D and Polycystic Ovary Syndrome (PCOS) reveals significant implications. Vitamin D deficiency, prevalent in PCOS, is closely tied to symptoms such as central obesity, IR, infertility, and hirsutism. Functioning as a steroid hormone with progesterone-like activity, vitamin D is pivotal in insulin synthesis, receptor expression, and glucose transport, normalizing calcium and parathyroid levels [31, 32, 40–42].

Supplementation studies suggest potential relief for PCOS symptoms, with observed reductions in total testosterone levels. Combining calcium and vitamin D enhances insulin levels, reduces resistance, and improves lipid profiles. A combination of metformin, calcium, and vitamin D exhibits positive impacts on weight loss, menstrual regularity, and hyperandrogenism in PCOS-associated infertility, with a noteworthy dose of 20,000 IU cholecalciferol weekly showcasing improvements in carbohydrate metabolism and menstrual frequency [31, 32, 41–43].

6.3.3 Zinc

Zinc is crucial for corpus luteum formation, supporting progesterone production essential for implantation [44]. Studies link zinc supplementation to elevated progesterone, while deficiency inhibits LH and estrogen, impacting luteal function [45–48]. Zinc supplementation is linked to enhanced lipid and glucose metabolism [32]. In an 8-week trial among PCOS women, zinc supplementation (50 mg elemental zinc/day) increased serum zinc and reduced IR, total cholesterol, LDL-C, triglycerides, testosterone, and TG/HDL-C ratio [49]. A study among PCOS subjects revealed that twice-daily co-supplementation of 250 mg magnesium oxide and 220 mg zinc sulphate (50 mg elemental zinc) notably decreased inflammation and oxidative stress markers [50]. These findings suggest potential benefits of at least 50 mg zinc/day for 8 weeks in PCOS management.

6.3.4 Selenium

As an antioxidant, selenium intake in PCOS may offer benefits by reducing oxidative stress along with IR, and hyperandrogenism, with its levels correlating with estrogen changes during the menstrual cycle [32, 51–57].

A rat model suggests that combined selenium nanoparticles and metformin therapy improve insulin sensitivity, lipid profile, inflammation, oxidative stress, and mitochondrial functions [51]. In different randomized trials, 200 μg daily selenium supplementation for 8–12 weeks in PCOS women showed improved pregnancy rates, reduced alopecia, acne, and lowered inflammatory markers [52–54]. Hence, a daily dose of 200 μg selenium for at least 8 weeks may benefit individuals with PCOS, suggesting potential advantages for hormonal and metabolic aspects, but it warrants further exploration.

6.3.5 Vitamin C

Vitamin C exhibits antioxidant properties and is involved in ovarian regulation and endometrial health. Vitamin C levels modulate throughout the menstrual cycle, affecting ovulation and progesterone production. Vitamin C levels decline immediately before ovulation and increase again after post-ovulation temperature rises. Ascorbic acid stimulates progesterone and oxytocin production. Vitamin C may play a role in regulating menstrual cycle irregularities in PCOS women, but further research is needed [40].

6.3.6 Vitamin E

Vitamin E, a crucial antioxidant, shows potential in counteracting reproductive system oxidative stress, impacting oocyte quality and countering pregnancy-related diseases [58]. It might positively affect endometrial thickness and overall ovarian function. Vitamin E supplementation, combined with coenzyme Q10, can increase SHBG levels and reduce free plasma testosterone concentrations in PCOS patients [40].

In a clinical trial with PCOS women, a 100 mg/day short-term vitamin E supplementation demonstrated the potential to diminish oxidative stress, resulting in reduced markers. Vitamin E can reduce oxidative stress, consequently reducing the exogenous human menopausal gonadotropin (HMG) dosage. The study revealed improved endometrial thickness and estrogen levels. However, this supplementation had no significant impact on pregnancy rates, regardless of initiation in the follicular or luteal phase [40, 58].

6.3.7 Inositol

Inositol represents a cyclic carbohydrate with six hydroxyl groups, one on each of the ring carbons. Nine stereoisomers of inositol exist, with myo-inositol (MI) and D-chiro-inositol (DCI) being the two primary stereoisomers found in the human body [40, 59, 60].

In the ovary, DCI plays a role in insulin-driven testosterone production, whereas MI is involved in FSH signaling. The insulin-dependent epimerase activity controls the ratio of MI to DCI, and it is noteworthy that ovaries do not develop IR, unlike muscles and the liver. This suggests that in PCOS, there could be an increased conversion of MI to DCI within the ovary due to insulin overproduction, resulting in excessive DCI levels and MI deficiency, disrupting hormonal balance [61].

6.3.8 Berberine

Berberine is a quaternary ammonium salt found in various medicinal plants like *Berberis and Hydrastis canadensis.* It belongs to the protoberberine group of isoquinoline alkaloids [62, 63]. Among PCOS patients, berberine positively impacts lipid profile, enhances insulin sensitivity, and increases ovulation rates, promoting fertility. It is considered safe for premenopausal women with minimal side effects [64]. It is efficient against IR and obesity, particularly targeting visceral adipose tissue [64], and if associated with a healthy lifestyle, improves women's body composition and causes androgen reduction [65]. Berberine may benefit PCOS management by improving metabolic, hormonal, and anthropometric parameters.

6.3.9 Polyphenols

Polyphenols, diverse secondary plant metabolites, are polyhydroxyphenols with multiple phenolic rings, often conjugated with sugars lacking nitrogen-based functional groups. Derived from shikimate and acetate pathways, they include phenolic acids, stilbenes, flavonoids, and lignans [66–68].

Resveratrol, a polyphenol found in grapes and berries, has anti-inflammatory and antioxidant properties. Initially considered for infertility treatment, caution is urged during pregnancy and the luteal phase due to potential adverse effects. Despite limitations, resveratrol inhibits proinflammatory cytokines, emphasizing the need for further PCOS research [40]. Various clinical trials using 800–1500 mg/day of resveratrol at least 40 days to 3 months have demonstrated positive effects on ovarian morphology, dominant follicle incidence, and androgen levels, anti-inflammatory effects and ER stress modulation, improved menstrual cyclicity and reduced hair loss in PCOS women [69–72]. Thus, resveratrol supplementation among PCOS women at doses up to 1500 mg/day for at least 40 days can be beneficial.

Naringenin, a key flavonoid in human diets, imparts color and a bitter-sour taste to foods. Found in grapefruit, sour orange, cherries, tomatoes, citrus fruits, and Greek oregano, it is also present in smaller amounts in bergamot, beans, fenugreek, milk thistle, tea, coffee, cocoa, and red wine naringenin's potential in PCOS treatment involves the AKT pathway, steroidogenesis, and gut microbiota modulation [73–75]. This indicates the supplementation of naringenin among PCOS women may be beneficial, but further study is required.

Quercetin, a flavonoid in fruits and vegetables, demonstrated therapeutic effects in PCOS treatment [76]. Administered at varying doses (15–150 mg/kg) for 3–10 weeks in rat models, it alleviated obesity, diabetes, and infertility. Quercetin enhanced antioxidants, reduced weight gain, normalized hormone levels, and inhibited PI3 kinase, showcasing multifaceted benefits in PCOS management [77–79]. A 40-day study with 500 mg quercetin supplementation among women daily reduced LH, TNF-alpha, and IL-6 levels, improved oocyte and embryo grades and increased pregnancy rates [80]. Thus, at least 500 mg/day supplementation of quercetin can be beneficial.

Individualized approach: supplementation needs vary among individuals, requiring consultation and active participation for optimal outcomes. A balanced diet and healthy lifestyle remain fundamental in PCOS therapy.

6.4 Herbs supporting treatment for PCOS

A balanced diet is vital in managing PCOS, and herbal extracts like Aloe vera, cinnamon, green tea, chamomile, and white mulberry complement this therapy. Certain herbs can influence lipid profiles, blood glucose, and IR, benefiting all PCOS phenotypes. Some herbs, such as green tea and marjoram, possess endocrine properties, improving hormonal levels, ovarian health, insulin sensitivity, and reducing inflammation. Green mint and liquorice root are recommended for women with elevated androgen levels. They have antiandrogen effects and reduce excess testosterone. Flaxseed lignans, turmeric, nettle, milk thistle, artichoke, dandelion, and black cumin offer various therapeutic benefits for PCOS, including antioxidant, anti-inflammatory, and hepatoprotective properties [32].

6.4.1 Flaxseed

Flaxseed, a nutrient-rich seed encompasses omega-3 fatty acids, lignans, fiber, niacin, vitamin E (39.5–50 mg/100 g), minerals, proteins, and peptides. With 37–45% lipid content, it is a prime omega-3 source. Rich in lignans and phenolic compounds, it offers diverse health benefits, including cardiovascular and anti-inflammatory effects [81, 82]. Flaxseed lignans stand out as well-studied dietary phytoestrogens. They can influence key enzymes involved in estrogen synthesis, shaping sex hormone levels [32]. A 4-month study on PCOS, patients taking 30 g/day of flaxseed exhibited reduced BMI, testosterone, insulin levels, and hirsutism [83]. In a 12-week study on women with PCOS, twice-daily supplementation of flaxseed oil omega-3 fatty acids (1000 mg capsule) significantly improved insulin levels, IR, hirsutism, triglycerides, VLDL-cholesterol, and CRP levels, demonstrating positive effects on insulin metabolism and specific metabolic markers [84]. Thus flaxseed (at least 20 g/day) or flaxseed oil flaxseed oil omega-3 fatty acids (1000 mg) for a minimum of 3 months can be beneficial for PCOS women.

6.4.2 Curcumin

Curcumin, found in turmeric, possesses strong antioxidant properties, reducing oxidative stress in PCOS patients. It also modulates proangiogenic and proinflammatory factors, suggesting potential pharmacologic benefits for PCOS [32, 85]. Turmeric extract exhibits promising effects in treating PCOS in albino rats, showing improvements in hormone and lipid profiles, antioxidant and glycaemic status, and ovarian morphology compared to metformin [85]. Additionally, in a mouse model, curcumin protects granulosa cells from apoptosis in PCOS rats by inhibiting the ER stress-related IRE1α-XBP1 pathway and activating the PI3K/AKT signaling pathway, suggesting its potential as a beneficial supplement for PCOS patients [86].

In a 12-week double-blind trial, curcumin intake (500 mg thrice daily) by women with PCOS demonstrated significant reductions in blood sugar and dehydroepiandrosterone, along with a potential increase in oestradiol [87]. Similarly, another study for 12 weeks found intake of 500 mg of curcumin per day can have beneficial effects on body weight, glycaemic control, and serum lipids except triglycerides and VLDL-cholesterol levels [88]. Most of the clinical trials using curcumin extract have used about 500–1500 mg of curcumin per day for 6–12 weeks has shown beneficial effects on PCOS patients [87–89].

6.4.3 Cinnamon

Cinnamon, valued for its fragrance, has diverse uses. Its essential oil, containing cinnamaldehyde, and the bark, with antioxidants like procyanidins, provide various biological benefits. The bark, rich in cinnamaldehyde, eugenol, and linalool, plays a significant role in its effects. With an abundance of phytochemicals, cinnamon exhibits potential health benefits, including anti-inflammatory, antimicrobial, antioxidant, and cardioprotective effects [90, 91].

A study done in mice found cinnamon (10 mg/100 g body weight) could restore oestrous cyclicity, normalize hormone levels, and improve ovarian morphology [92]. A 12-week study among women with PCOS using cinnamon powder capsules (1.5 g/day in three doses) showed significant reductions in fasting insulin and IR, with a decrease in low-density lipoprotein levels [93]. Thus, about 1.5 g of cinnamon powder consumption can be beneficial for PCOS women.

7. Lifestyle in PCOS management

7.1 Exercise and physical activity in PCOS management

Exercise offers metabolic benefits beyond weight management, particularly relevant to PCOS-related risk factors like hypertension, IR, elevated blood glucose, and endothelial dysfunction. Research demonstrates that increased physical activity and fitness, regardless of weight loss, can ameliorate these factors. Endurance training has been shown to reduce IR and improve metabolic profiles in overweight PCOS women. Combining aerobic and resistance training proves effective in reducing IR and body fat, and resistance training maintains basal metabolic rate and enhances muscle strength, facilitating regular physical activity [29].

Exercise reduces IR by two mechanisms as below [30]:

- Induces a reduction in visceral fat even if there is moderate weight loss and BMI reduction.
- Increases muscle cell metabolism: Exercise modulates the expression or the activity of proteins mediating insulin signaling in the skeletal muscles.

It has been shown that exercise improves menstrual abnormalities and restores ovulation in obese patients with PCOS, and its benefit on reproductive function is greater than the benefit of a low-calorie diet only. Exercise exerts its beneficial effects on body composition with greater reduction in fat mass and better preservation of fat-free mass [30]. Collectively, the evidence underscores the health advantages of exercise, both for weight management and metabolic well-being in PCOS and beyond [29].

Exercise is increasingly recognized as a vital element in managing PCOS, enhancing insulin sensitivity through optimized glucose transport and metabolism. Recent research emphasizes the importance of exercise intensity for health improvements. Meta-analysis and systematic reviews highlight the significant impact of vigorous intensity exercise on factors like cardiorespiratory fitness, IR, and body composition. Studies using metrics like HOMA-IR and BMI show substantial decreases in IR, supporting the benefits of physical activity. Engaging in a minimum of 120 minutes of aerobic activity per week is recommended for optimal results in managing PCOS-related concerns [32].

Public health recommendations advise overweight and obese individuals, including those with PCOS, to gradually increase physical activity to 200–300 minutes per week of moderate exercise, like brisk walking, to prevent unhealthy weight regain and promote long-term weight maintenance. This evidence highlights the importance of incorporating adequate physical activity into PCOS weight management programmes [29]. At the moment, there are no guidelines for the type, intensity, frequency, and duration of exercise in patients with PCOS, but physical activities as of a normal adult should performed regularly as below [30]:

- *Moderate-intensity aerobic physical activity* (e.g., brisk walking) for at least 30 min and for at least 5 days per week should be recommended in all PCOS patients.
- *Vigorous-intensity aerobic activity* (e.g., jogging) for at least 20 min and for at least 3 days per week or combinations of moderate- and vigorous-intensity exercise can also be recommended.

- *Resistance training* for at least two non-consecutive days per week.
- *Endurance exercise* for patients who cannot manage high-intensity exercise, prolonged lower-level activity is an appropriate way to gain fitness and increase energy expenditure (**Table 2**).

7.2 Lifestyle modification

Lifestyle intervention (diet and physical activity) leading to a 5–10% weight loss has shown significant improvements in IR, ovulation, menstrual regularity, and other PCOS symptoms. Women with PCOS adopt both healthy and non-healthy practices for weight management. Despite its benefits, many PCOS patients do not receive lifestyle advice from healthcare providers. Lifestyle programmes combine diet, exercise, and cognitive strategies. They have been effective in preventing diabetes and improving PCOS-related factors like weight, hormones, and metabolic issues. Studies support their impact on BMI, blood glucose, and hormonal balance. While positive effects are seen, clinical reproductive outcomes and quality of life need further study. Combining lifestyle changes with treatments like metformin can enhance results. In overweight PCOS women, lifestyle changes led to better menstrual regularity and insulin sensitivity. Lifestyle interventions should be the primary approach for PCOS management, but maintaining healthy habits long-term remains a challenge. A team-based approach could offer better results for comprehensive PCOS care [31].

1. Support from health professional, family, spouse, peers is necessary for lifestyle modification.
2. Prioritize smoking cessation and reduce alcohol consumption.
3. Weight loss/maintenance and lifestyle modification programmes should be well structured and individualized according to health professionals' advice.
4. Summary of the main components of exercise prescription based on *FITT*:
    - *Frequency*: engage in physical activity 3–5 days per week, emphasizing the establishment of a consistent exercise routine before advancing frequency.
    - *Intensity*: initiate with low to moderate intensity, gradually increasing over weeks, prioritizing duration for optimal energy expenditure, emphasizing prolonged activity over intensity.
    - *Time*: 30–60 min, using a gradual progression (can be accumulated in multiple short bouts of at least 10 min that may promote greater adherence).
    - *Type*: choose low-impact activities such as walking, cycling, or low-impact aerobics, ensuring convenience and enjoyment.
5. *Resistance training*: should be performed two to three times per week, with one set of 8–15 repetitions at a moderate intensity, using 8–10 different exercises that work each of the major muscle groups.
6. *Warm-up and cool-down*: emphasize appropriate warm-up and cool-down periods to enhance safety and flexibility.
7. *Daily lifestyle activities*: emphasize reducing sedentary behaviors and time spent being physically inactive. Increase participation in daily lifestyle activities such as stair climbing, walking during breaks, climbing stairs whenever possible, and house cleaning.

Adapted from: Refs. [30, 39].

Table 2.
Exercise and lifestyle modification guidelines.

Exercise is a vital component of successful lifestyle modifications for weight management in PCOS. Studies show that physical activity is associated with sustained weight loss and that combining exercise with diet enhances weight reduction compared to diet alone. Research suggests that highly active individuals have the greatest success in maintaining weight loss [29].

Lifestyle adjustments play a crucial role in managing PCOS in women, complementing medical treatments. This encompasses regular behavioral adjustments, social support, and psychological adaptations. Essential modifications include maintaining regular physical activity and exercise, long-term weight management strategy, adhering to a balanced diet, behavior therapies, and avoiding tobacco—a comprehensive approach aligned with clinical guidelines to prevent and treat metabolic issues. Prioritizing overall well-being and mental health is a personal choice, offering valuable steps toward a more fulfilling life [29, 32].

8. Conclusion

Polycystic Ovary Syndrome (PCOS) is a complex endocrine disorder affecting women, marked by hormonal imbalances, menstrual irregularities, and ovarian cysts. Its pathophysiology involves genetic, environmental, and hormonal factors, disrupting the HPO axis and contributing to reproductive and metabolic complexities. Hyperandrogenism, ovarian dysfunction, insulin resistance, and obesity amplify PCOS's intricacy, elevating the risk of metabolic syndrome and cardiovascular diseases. The interplay of genetic predisposition and an "obesogenic" environment remains to be fully elucidated. PCOS complications encompass menstrual irregularities, hirsutism, acne, alopecia, acanthosis nigricans, dyslipidaemia, fatty liver disease, inflammation, obstructive sleep apnoea, gestational diabetes, type II diabetes, infertility, and recurrent pregnancy loss.

PCOS management includes supplementation with vitamin D, zinc, selenium, omega-3 fatty acids, vitamin C, vitamin E, chromium, inositol, and berberine. These supplements address deficiencies, reduce inflammation, improve hormonal balance, enhance insulin sensitivity, and mitigate metabolic abnormalities in PCOS patients. An individualized approach, considering diverse needs and factors, is essential for optimal outcomes, emphasizing the importance of a balanced diet and a healthy lifestyle in PCOS therapy. Further research is needed to establish precise dosages and guidelines for supplementation in PCOS management.

Polyphenols like resveratrol, naringenin, and rutin show antioxidant benefits. Herbs such as flaxseed, turmeric, nettle, and traditional remedies offer diverse therapeutic support for PCOS management. Exercise, particularly aerobic and resistance training, plays a crucial role in managing PCOS. It improves insulin sensitivity, reproductive function, and overall health, promoting lasting lifestyle changes.

Personalized, sustainable lifestyle adjustments, including 5–10% weight loss, significantly improve PCOS symptoms, enhancing IR, ovulation, and menstrual regularity. A team-based approach could offer better results for comprehensive PCOS care. A holistic approach to PCOS management involves medical treatments complemented by lifestyle modification, which integrates exercise, dietary adjustments, and prioritizing psychological well-being for comprehensive women's health.

DOI: http://dx.doi.org/10.5772/intechopen.114149

Conflict of interest

The authors declare no conflict of interest.

Author details

Madan Pandey[1]* and Kritee Niroula[2]

1 Metro Kathmandu Hospital, Kathmandu, Nepal

2 Central Campus of Technology, Tribhuvan University, Dharan, Nepal

*Address all correspondence to: cumyps23@gmail.com

References

[1] Rosenberg SL. The relationship between PCOS and obesity: Which comes first? The Science Journal of the Lander College of Arts and Sciences. 2019;**13**(1):5

[2] Ndefo UA, Eaton A, Green MR. Polycystic ovary syndrome: A review of treatment options with a focus on pharmacological approaches. P & T: A Peer-reviewed Journal for Formulary Management. 2013;**38**(6):336-355

[3] Stracquadanio M, Ciotta L. Introduction. In: Stracquadanio M, Ciotta L, editors. Metabolic Aspects of PCOS: Treatment with Insulin Sensitizers. Cham: Springer International Publishing; 2015. pp. 1-4

[4] Zeng X, Xie Y-j, Liu Y-t, Long S-l, Mo Z-c. Polycystic ovarian syndrome: Correlation between hyperandrogenism, insulin resistance and obesity. Clinica Chimica Acta. 2020;**502**:214-221

[5] Di Pietro M, Pascuali N, Parborell F, Abramovich D. Ovarian angiogenesis in polycystic ovary syndrome. Reproduction. 2018;**155**(5):R199-R209

[6] Teede HJ, Misso ML, Deeks AA, Moran LJ, Stuckey BGA, Wong JLA, et al. Assessment and management of polycystic ovary syndrome: Summary of an evidence-based guideline. Medical Journal of Australia. 2011;**195**(S6):S65-S112

[7] McGee EA, Hsueh AJW. Initial and cyclic recruitment of ovarian follicles*. Endocrine Reviews. 2000;**21**(2):200-214

[8] Luderer U. Ovarian toxicity from reactive oxygen species. Vitamins and Hormones. 2014;**94**:99-127

[9] Wallace WH, Kelsey TW. Human ovarian reserve from conception to the menopause. PLoS One. 2010;**5**(1):e8772

[10] Findlay JK, Hutt KJ, Hickey M, Anderson RA. How is the number of primordial follicles in the ovarian reserve established? Biology of Reproduction. 2015;**93**(5):1-7

[11] Dumont A, Robin G, Catteau-Jonard S, Dewailly D. Role of anti-Müllerian hormone in pathophysiology, diagnosis and treatment of polycystic ovary syndrome: A review. Reproductive Biology and Endocrinology. 2015;**13**(1):137

[12] Ibáñez L, Oberfield Sharon E, Witchel S, Auchus Richard J, Chang RJ, Codner E, et al. An international consortium update: Pathophysiology, diagnosis, and treatment of polycystic ovarian syndrome in adolescence. Hormone Research in Paediatrics. 2017;**88**(6):371-395

[13] Stracquadanio M, Ciotta L. Etiopathogenesis. In: Stracquadanio M, Ciotta L, editors. Metabolic Aspects of PCOS: Treatment with Insulin Sensitizers. Cham: Springer International Publishing; 2015. pp. 5-20

[14] Rudnicka E, Kunicki M, Calik-Ksepka A, Suchta K, Duszewska A, Smolarczyk K, et al. Anti-Müllerian hormone in pathogenesis, diagnostic and treatment of PCOS. International Journal of Molecular Sciences. 2021;**22**(22):12507

[15] Witchel SF, Oberfield SE, Peña AS. Polycystic ovary syndrome: Pathophysiology, presentation, and treatment with emphasis on adolescent girls. Journal of the Endocrine Society. 2019;**3**(8):1545-1573

[16] Balen A. The pathophysiology of polycystic ovary syndrome: Trying to understand PCOS and its endocrinology. Best Practice & Research Clinical Obstetrics & Gynaecology. 2004;**18**(5):685-706

[17] Goodarzi MO, Dumesic DA, Chazenbalk G, Azziz R. Polycystic ovary syndrome: Etiology, pathogenesis and diagnosis. Nature Reviews Endocrinology. 2011;**7**(4):219-231

[18] Sanchez-Garrido MA, Tena-Sempere M. Metabolic dysfunction in polycystic ovary syndrome: Pathogenic role of androgen excess and potential therapeutic strategies. Molecular Metabolism. 2020;**35**:100937

[19] Glueck CJ, Goldenberg N. Characteristics of obesity in polycystic ovary syndrome: Etiology, treatment, and genetics. Metabolism. 2019;**92**:108-120

[20] Stracquadanio M, Ciotta L. Clinical features. In: Stracquadanio M, Ciotta L, editors. Metabolic Aspects of PCOS: Treatment with Insulin Sensitizers. Cham: Springer International Publishing; 2015. pp. 21-62

[21] Johnston-MacAnanny EB, Berga SL. Polycystic ovary syndrome. In: Falcone T, Hurd WW, editors. Clinical reproductive medicine and surgery: A practical guide. Cham: Springer International Publishing; 2017. pp. 123-137

[22] Paschou SA, Polyzos SA, Anagnostis P, Goulis DG, Kanaka-Gantenbein C, Lambrinoudaki I, et al. Nonalcoholic fatty liver disease in women with polycystic ovary syndrome. Endocrine. 2020;**67**(1):1-8

[23] de Melo AS, Dias SV, Cavalli RC, Cardoso VC, Bettiol H, Barbieri MA, et al. Pathogenesis of polycystic ovary syndrome: Multifactorial assessment from the foetal stage to menopause. Reproduction. 2015;**150**(1):R11-R24

[24] Puttabyatappa M, Padmanabhan V. Ovarian and extra-ovarian mediators in the development of polycystic ovary syndrome. Journal of Molecular Endocrinology. 2018;**61**(4):R161-RR84

[25] Goyal A, Ganie MA. Idiopathic hyperprolactinemia presenting as polycystic ovary syndrome in identical twin sisters: A case report and literature review. Cureus. 2018;**10**(7):e3004

[26] Spinedi E, Cardinali DP. The polycystic ovary syndrome and the metabolic syndrome: A possible chronobiotic-cytoprotective adjuvant therapy. International Journal of Endocrinology. 2018;**2018**:1349868

[27] Albu D, Albu A. The relationship between anti-Müllerian hormone serum level and body mass index in a large cohort of infertile patients. Endocrine. 2019;**63**(1):157-163

[28] Rosenfield RL, Ehrmann DA. The pathogenesis of polycystic ovary syndrome (PCOS): The hypothesis of PCOS as functional ovarian hyperandrogenism revisited. Endocrine Reviews. 2016;**37**(5):467-520

[29] Moran LJ, Brinkworth GD, Norman RJ. Dietary therapy in polycystic ovary syndrome. Seminars in Reproductive Medicine. 2008;**26**(01):085-092

[30] Stracquadanio M, Ciotta L. PCOS therapy. In: Stracquadanio M, Ciotta L, editors. Metabolic Aspects of PCOS: Treatment with Insulin Sensitizers. Cham: Springer International Publishing; 2015. pp. 89-137

[31] Papavasiliou K, Papakonstantinou E. Nutritional support and dietary

interventions for women with polycystic ovary syndrome. Nutrition and Dietary Supplements. 2017;**9**:63-85

[32] Szczuko M, Kikut J, Szczuko U, Szydłowska I, Nawrocka-Rutkowska J, Ziętek M, et al. Nutrition strategy and life style in polycystic ovary syndrome—Narrative review. Nutrients. 2021;**13**(7):2452

[33] Szczuko M, Szydłowska I, Nawrocka-Rutkowska J. A properly balanced reduction diet and/or supplementation solve the problem with the deficiency of these vitamins soluble in water in patients with PCOS. Nutrients. 2021;**13**(3):2-10

[34] Esmaeilzadeh S, Gholinezhad-Chari M, Ghadimi R. The effect of metformin treatment on the serum levels of homocysteine, folic acid, and vitamin B12 in patients with polycystic ovary syndrome. Journal of Human Reproductive Sciences. 2017;**10**(2):95-101

[35] Zaeemzadeh N, Jahanian Sadatmahalleh S, Ziaei S, Kazemnejad A, Movahedinejad M, Mottaghi A, et al. Comparison of dietary micronutrient intake in PCOS patients with and without metabolic syndrome. Journal of Ovarian Research. 2021;**14**(1):10

[36] Tripathi S, Singh M, Jain M, Khatoon S. Nutritional perspective of polycystic ovarian syndrome: A review study. Current Medicine Research and Practice. 2020;**10**(2):65-69

[37] Neves LPP, Marcondes RR, Maffazioli GDN, Simões RS, Maciel GAR, Soares JM, et al. Nutritional and dietary aspects in polycystic ovary syndrome: Insights into the biology of nutritional interventions. Gynecological Endocrinology. 2020;**36**(12):1047-1050

[38] Zhang X, Zheng Y, Guo Y, Lai Z. The effect of low carbohydrate diet on polycystic ovary syndrome: A meta-analysis of randomized controlled trials. International Journal of Endocrinology. 2019;**2019**:4386401

[39] Moran LJ, Brinkworth G, Noakes M, Norman RJ. Effects of lifestyle modification in polycystic ovarian syndrome. Reproductive Biomedicine Online. 2006;**12**(5):569-578

[40] Iervolino M, Lepore E, Forte G, Laganà AS, Buzzaccarini G, Unfer V. Natural molecules in the Management of Polycystic Ovary Syndrome (PCOS): An analytical review. Nutrients. 2021;**13**(5):1677

[41] Teegarden D, Donkin SS. Vitamin D: Emerging new roles in insulin sensitivity. Nutrition Research Reviews. 2009;**22**(1):82-92

[42] He C, Lin Z, Robb SW, Ezeamama AE. Serum vitamin D levels and polycystic ovary syndrome: A systematic review and meta-analysis. Nutrients. 2015;**7**(6):4555-4577

[43] Wehr E, Pieber TR, Obermayer-Pietsch B. Effect of vitamin D3 treatment on glucose metabolism and menstrual frequency in polycystic ovary syndrome women: A pilot study. Journal of Endocrinological Investigation. 2011;**34**(10):757-763

[44] Sunar F, Baltaci AK, Ergene N, Mogulkoc R. Zinc deficiency and supplementation in ovariectomized rats: Their effect on serum estrogen and progesterone levels and their relation to calcium and phosphorus. Pakistan Journal of Pharmaceutical Sciences. 2009;**22**(2):150-154

[45] Kechrid Z, Amamra S, Bouzerna N. The effect of zinc deficiency on zinc

status, carbohydrate metabolism and progesterone level in pregnant rats. Turkish Journal of Medical Sciences. 2006;**36**(6):337-342

[46] Om AS, Chung KW. Dietary zinc deficiency alters 5 alpha-reduction and aromatization of testosterone and androgen and estrogen receptors in rat liver. The Journal of Nutrition. 1996;**126**(4):842-848

[47] Humeny A, Bökenkamp D, Thole HH. The HDQVH-motif in domain E of the estradiol receptor alpha is responsible for zinc-binding and zinc-induced hormone release. Molecular and Cellular Endocrinology. 1999;**153**(1-2):71-78

[48] Noda Y, Ota K, Shirasawa T, Shimizu T. Copper/zinc superoxide dismutase insufficiency impairs progesterone secretion and fertility in female Mice1. Biology of Reproduction. 2012;**86**(1):1-8

[49] Pourteymourfard TF, Alipour B, Mehrzad SM, Ostad RA. Effect of zinc supplementation on cardiometabolic risk factors in women with polycystic ovary syndrome. Journal of Cardiovascular and Thoracic Research. 2010;**2**(2):11-20

[50] Afshar Ebrahimi F, Foroozanfard F, Aghadavod E, Bahmani F, Asemi Z. The effects of magnesium and zinc co-supplementation on biomarkers of inflammation and oxidative stress, and gene expression related to inflammation in polycystic ovary syndrome: A randomized controlled clinical trial. Biological Trace Element Research. 2018;**184**(2):300-307

[51] Rabah HM, Mohamed DA, Mariah RA, Abd El-Khalik SR, Khattab HA, AbuoHashish NA, et al. Novel insights into the synergistic effects of selenium nanoparticles and metformin treatment of letrozole-induced polycystic ovarian syndrome: Targeting PI3K/Akt signalling pathway, redox status and mitochondrial dysfunction in ovarian tissue. Redox Report. 2023;**28**(1):2160569

[52] Razavi M, Jamilian M, Kashan ZF, Heidar Z, Mohseni M, Ghandi Y, et al. Selenium supplementation and the effects on reproductive outcomes, biomarkers of inflammation, and oxidative stress in women with polycystic ovary syndrome. Horm Metab Res = Hormone and metabolic research = Hormon- und Stoffwechselforschung = Hormones et metabolisme. 2016;**48**(3):185-190

[53] Jamilian M, Razavi M, Fakhrie Kashan Z, Ghandi Y, Bagherian T, Asemi Z. Metabolic response to selenium supplementation in women with polycystic ovary syndrome: A randomized, double-blind, placebo-controlled trial. Clinical Endocrinology. 2015;**82**(6):885-891

[54] Rashidi BH, Mohammad Hosseinzadeh F, Alipoor E, Asghari S, Yekaninejad MS, Hosseinzadeh-Attar MJ. Effects of selenium supplementation on asymmetric dimethylarginine and cardiometabolic risk factors in patients with polycystic ovary syndrome. Biological Trace Element Research. 2020;**196**(2):430-437

[55] Zhao J, Dong L, Lin Z, Sui X, Wang Y, Li L, et al. Effects of selenium supplementation on polycystic ovarian syndrome: A systematic review and meta-analysis on randomized clinical trials. BMC Endocrine Disorders. 2023;**23**(1):33

[56] Hajizadeh-Sharafabad F, Moludi J, Tutunchi H, Taheri E, Izadi A, Maleki V. Selenium and polycystic ovary syndrome; current knowledge and future directions: A systematic review.

Hormone and Metabolism Research. 2019;**51**(05):279-287

[57] Pieczyńska J, Grajeta H. The role of selenium in human conception and pregnancy. Journal of Trace Elements in Medicine and Biology. 2015;**29**:31-38

[58] Chen J, Guo Q, Pei YH, Ren QL, Chi L, Hu RK, et al. Effect of a short-term vitamin E supplementation on oxidative stress in infertile PCOS women under ovulation induction: A retrospective cohort study. BMC Women's Health. 2020;**20**(1):69

[59] Caputo M, Bona E, Leone I, Samà MT, Nuzzo A, Ferrero A, et al. Inositols and metabolic disorders: From farm to bedside. Journal of Traditional and Complementary Medicine. 2020;**10**(3):252-259

[60] Murthy PPN. Structure and nomenclature of inositol phosphates, phosphoinositides, and glycosylphosphatidylinositols. In: Majumder AL, Biswas BB, editors. Biology of Inositols and Phosphoinositides: Subcellular Biochemistry. Boston, MA: Springer US; 2006. pp. 1-19

[61] Facchinetti F, Bizzarri M, Benvenga S, D'Anna R, Lanzone A, Soulage C, et al. Results from the international consensus conference on Myo-inositol and d-chiro-inositol in obstetrics and gynecology: The link between metabolic syndrome and PCOS. European Journal of Obstetrics, Gynecology, and Reproductive Biology. 2015;**195**:72-76

[62] Zhang S-w, Zhou J, Gober H-J, Leung WT, Wang L. Effect and mechanism of berberine against polycystic ovary syndrome. Biomedicine & Pharmacotherapy. 2021;**138**:111468

[63] Cicero AFG, Baggioni A. Berberine and its role in chronic disease. In: Gupta SC, Prasad S, Aggarwal BB, editors. Anti-Inflammatory Nutraceuticals and Chronic Diseases. Cham: Springer International Publishing; 2016. pp. 27-45

[64] Rondanelli M, Infantino V, Riva A, Petrangolini G, Faliva MA, Peroni G, et al. Polycystic ovary syndrome management: A review of the possible amazing role of berberine. Archives of Gynecology and Obstetrics. 2020;**301**(1):53-60

[65] Saleem F, Rizvi SW. New therapeutic approaches in obesity and metabolic syndrome associated with polycystic ovary syndrome. Cureus. 2017;**9**(11):e1844

[66] Quideau S, Deffieux D, Douat-Casassus C, Pouységu L. Plant polyphenols: Chemical properties, biological activities, and synthesis. Angewandte Chemie, International Edition. 2011;**50**(3):586-621

[67] Bravo L. Polyphenols: Chemistry, dietary sources, metabolism, and nutritional significance. Nutrition Reviews. 1998;**56**(11):317-333

[68] Spencer JPE, Abd El Mohsen MM, Minihane A-M, Mathers JC. Biomarkers of the intake of dietary polyphenols: Strengths, limitations and application in nutrition research. British Journal of Nutrition. 2008;**99**(1):12-22

[69] Hashemi Taheri AP, Moradi B, Radmard AR, Sanginabadi M, Qorbani M, Mohajeri-Tehrani MR, et al. Effect of resveratrol administration on ovarian morphology, determined by transvaginal ultrasound for the women with polycystic ovary syndrome (PCOS). British Journal of Nutrition. 2022;**128**(2):211-216

[70] Banaszewska B, Wrotyńska-Barczyńska J, Spaczynski RZ,

Pawelczyk L, Duleba AJ. Effects of resveratrol on polycystic ovary syndrome: A double-blind, randomized, placebo-controlled trial. The Journal of Clinical Endocrinology & Metabolism. 2016;**101**(11):4322-4328

[71] Brenjian S, Moini A, Yamini N, Kashani L, Faridmojtahedi M, Bahramrezaie M, et al. Resveratrol treatment in patients with polycystic ovary syndrome decreased pro-inflammatory and endoplasmic reticulum stress markers. American Journal of Reproductive Immunology (New York, NY : 1989). 2020;**83**(1):e13186

[72] Mansour A, Samadi M, Sanginabadi M, Gerami H, Karimi S, Hosseini S, et al. Effect of resveratrol on menstrual cyclicity, hyperandrogenism and metabolic profile in women with PCOS. Clinical Nutrition (Edinburgh, Scotland). 2021;**40**(6):4106-4112

[73] Hong Y, Yin Y, Tan Y, Hong K, Zhou H. The flavanone, naringenin, modifies antioxidant and steroidogenic enzyme activity in a rat model of letrozole-induced polycystic ovary syndrome. Medical Science Monitor: International Medical Journal of Experimental and Clinical Research. 2019;**25**:395-401

[74] Wu Y-X, Yang X-Y, Han B-S, Hu Y-Y, An T, Lv B-H, et al. Naringenin regulates gut microbiota and SIRT1/ PGC-1α signaling pathway in rats with letrozole-induced polycystic ovary syndrome. Biomedicine & Pharmacotherapy. 2022;**153**:113286

[75] Rashid R, Tripathi R, Singh A, Sarkar S, Kawale A, Bader GN, et al. Naringenin improves ovarian health by reducing the serum androgen and eliminating follicular cysts in letrozole-induced polycystic ovary syndrome in the Sprague Dawley rats. Phytotherapy Research. 2023;**37**(9):4018-4041

[76] Luo E-D, Jiang H-M, Chen W, Wang Y, Tang M, Guo W-M, et al. Advancements in lead therapeutic phytochemicals polycystic ovary syndrome: A review. Frontiers in Pharmacology. 2023;**13**:1-21

[77] Jafari Khorchani M, Zal F, Neisy A. The phytoestrogen, quercetin, in serum, uterus and ovary as a potential treatment for dehydroepiandrosterone-induced polycystic ovary syndrome in the rat. Reproduction, Fertility, and Development. 2020;**32**(3):313-321

[78] Hong Y, Yin Y, Tan Y, Hong K, Jiang F, Wang Y. Effect of quercetin on biochemical parameters in letrozoleinduced polycystic ovary syndrome in rats. Tropical Journal of Pharmaceutical Research. 2018;**17**(9):1783-1788

[79] Shah KN, Patel SS. Phosphatidylinositide 3-kinase inhibition: A new potential target for the treatment of polycystic ovarian syndrome. Pharmaceutical Biology. 2016;**54**(6):975-983

[80] Vaez S, Parivr K, Amidi F, Rudbari NH, Moini A, Amini N. Quercetin and polycystic ovary syndrome; inflammation, hormonal parameters and pregnancy outcome: A randomized clinical trial. American Journal of Reproductive Immunology (New York, NY : 1989). 2023;**89**(3):e13644

[81] Nowak W, Jeziorek M. The Role of Flaxseed in Improving Human Health. Healthcare (Basel, Switzerland). 2023;11(3):1-20

[82] Kajla P, Sharma A, Sood DR. Flaxseed-a potential functional food source. Journal of Food Science and Technology. 2015;**52**(4):1857-1871

[83] Nowak DA, Snyder DC, Brown AJ, Demark-Wahnefried W. The effect of flaxseed supplementation on hormonal levels associated with polycystic ovarian syndrome: A case study. Current Topics in Nutraceutical Research. 2007;**5**(4):177-181

[84] Mirmasoumi G, Fazilati M, Foroozanfard F, Vahedpoor Z, Mahmoodi S, Taghizadeh M, et al. The effects of flaxseed oil Omega-3 fatty acids supplementation on metabolic status of patients with polycystic ovary syndrome: A randomized, double-blind, placebo-controlled trial. Experimental and Clinical Endocrinology & Diabetes: Official Journal, German Society of Endocrinology [and] German Diabetes Association. 2018;**126**(4):222-228

[85] Shah MZH, Shrivastava VK. Turmeric extract alleviates endocrine-metabolic disturbances in letrozole-induced PCOS by increasing adiponectin circulation: A comparison with metformin. Metabolism Open. 2022;**13**:100160

[86] Zhang Y, Wang L, Weng Y, Wang D, Wang R, Wang H, et al. Curcumin inhibits hyperandrogen-induced IRE1α-XBP1 pathway activation by activating the PI3K/AKT signaling in ovarian granulosa cells of PCOS model rats. Oxidative Medicine and Cellular Longevity. 2022;**2022**:20

[87] Heshmati J, Moini A, Sepidarkish M, Morvaridzadeh M, Salehi M, Palmowski A, et al. Effects of curcumin supplementation on blood glucose, insulin resistance and androgens in patients with polycystic ovary syndrome: A randomized double-blind placebo-controlled clinical trial. Phytomedicine. 2021;**80**:153395

[88] Jamilian M, Foroozanfard F, Kavossian E, Aghadavod E, Shafabakhsh R, Hoseini A, et al. Effects of curcumin on body weight, glycemic control and serum lipids in women with polycystic ovary syndrome: A randomized, double-blind, placebo-controlled trial. Clinical Nutrition ESPEN. 2020;**36**:128-133

[89] Jabczyk M, Nowak J, Hudzik B, Zubelewicz-Szkodzińska B. Curcumin in metabolic health and disease. Nutrients. 2021;**13**(12):4440

[90] Rao PV, Gan SH. Cinnamon: A multifaceted medicinal plant. Evidence-Based Complementary and Alternative Medicine. 2014;**2014**:642942

[91] Gruenwald J, Freder J, Armbruester N. Cinnamon and health. Critical Reviews in Food Science and Nutrition. 2010;**50**(9):822-834

[92] Dou L, Zheng Y, Li L, Gui X, Chen Y, Yu M, et al. The effect of cinnamon on polycystic ovary syndrome in a mouse model. Reproductive Biology and Endocrinology: RB&E. 2018;**16**(1):99

[93] Hajimonfarednejad M, Nimrouzi M, Heydari M, Zarshenas MM, Raee MJ, Jahromi BN. Insulin resistance improvement by cinnamon powder in polycystic ovary syndrome: A randomized double-blind placebo controlled clinical trial. Phytotherapy Research. 2018;**32**(2):276-283

Section 2

Polycystic Ovary Syndrome Causes

Chapter 3

Causes of Polycystic Ovarian Syndrome

Subrat Panda, Rituparna Das, Lisley Konar and Manasi Singh

Abstract

PCOS is a multifactorial syndromic disorder—the exact etiology is not known. Genetic, epigenetic, and environmental factors may be the causative factors. It is the most common cause of an-ovulatory infertility, and in adolescents, the young girl may present with irregular periods. Most of the women with PCOS are either overweight or obese. Another variety of PCOS women is lean. Sleep apnea, metabolic syndrome, and endometrial carcinoma are the late consequences of women with PCOS. As new research shows that gut microbiome is one of the attributing factors of PCOS, it will lead to a new horizon in the management of PCOS. Fecal implantation or probiotics may be helpful in PCOS management. Physical and emotional stress is one of the contributing factors to PCOS. Neuroendocrine factors are also an attributive factor for the development of PCOS. Most of the research about neuroendocrine factors is very preliminary and limited to the mice model. The incidence of PCOS varies from region to region as dietary and environmental factors differ. More human research is required to have more knowledge about the etiology of PCOS, which will guide the management of PCOS.

Keywords: PCOS, FSH, LH, EDC, SFA, ROS, Genomic variants, hyperandrogenism, NEFAs, SHBG, gut microbiome

1. Introduction

PCOS is a reproductive dysfunction resulting from an interaction between endocrine and metabolic disorders. Hyperandrogenism and insulin resistance complement one another in the development of PCOS. Primarily, it is affected by alteration of the hypothalamus-pituitary-ovarian axis. The cyclic pattern of hormone concentrations, which is the characteristic determinant of normal ovulatory menstrual cycles, is lost in women with PCOS. In these women, there is chronic anovulation resulting in a "steady low state" of gonadotropin and sex steroid concentrations. Daily production of both androgens and oestrogens is increased. Chronic hyperandrogenemia and insulin resistance (usually, though not always, associated with obesity) also result in ovarian dysfunction of PCOS. PCOS women suffer from oligomenorrhoea, infertility, metabolic syndrome, acne and oily skin, hirsutism, and endometrial carcinoma at a later age. The pathophysiology of PCOS is most likely multifactorial, involving endocrine, metabolic, genetic, epigenetic, and environmental factors. Increased serum luteinising hormone (LH) concentrations, low-normal follicle-stimulating hormone (FSH) levels and increased LH-to-FSH ratios is a feature of women with PCOS. Insulin resistance is usually seen in obese PCOS women and, to a lesser extent, in women with lean PCOS. In general, the prevalence varies from 50 and 75% [1]. About 35% of women with polycystic ovary syndrome exhibit impaired glucose tolerance, and up to 10% meet the criteria for type 2 diabetes mellitus. Insulin and LH act synergistically, resulting hyperandrogenism. Insulin resistance and hyperinsulinemia are the cause, not the result, of hyperandrogenism in PCOS. Women with PCOS have increased visceral fat than subcutaneous fat. Women with lean PCOS have an increased percentage of body fat, a higher waist–hip ratio, and greater intra-abdominal, peritoneal, and visceral fat compared to normal women matched for body mass index (BMI) [2]. Women with PCOS suffer from different psychological disorder. The diagnosis of PCOS is based on the 2003 Rotterdam criteria, where the incidence of two out of the three criteria hyperandrogenism (clinical and/or biochemical), irregular cycles, and polycystic ovary morphology. Evidence-based medicine suggests that the anti-Mullerian hormone in serum can be used as a substitute for the follicular count, and it is thereby emerging as an official polycystic ovarian morphology/PCOS marker. The limitation of this criteria is mainly in the diagnosis of adolescents as the features of PCOS overlap with the normal physiological change in puberty. Therefore, PCOM should not be considered a criterion in the first 8 years of menarche, and the essential criteria are irregular menstrual cycles and clinical and/or biochemical hyperandrogenism.

2. Genetic association

Familial aggregation studies identify PCOS as an inherited disorder. Higher frequency of genetic polymorphism at 2p16.3 (rs13405728), 2p21 (rs13429458), and 9q33.3 (rs2479106) are noted in women with PCOS. In one group of patients, X-linked inheritance was seen. Siblings and parents of patients suffering from PCOS have a high prevalence of hyperinsulinemia and hypertriglyceridemia, PCOS in females, and premature balding in males. Monozygotic twin sisters have twice the risk of developing PCOS. About 50% of sisters of patients with PCOS have increased levels of total or bioavailable testosterone concentrations, and 35% of their mothers also suffer from PCOS [3]. First-degree relatives of women with PCOS have features of metabolic syndrome. PCOS is described as a polygenic disorder that includes the interplay of various genomic variants (**Table 1**).

In pregnancy in PCOS mothers, there is placental dysfunction due to hyperinsulinemia leading to hyperandrogenic foetal micro-environment. The theory of hyperinsulinemia suggests that there are two factors involved: maternal insulin resistance and decreased placental aromatase, which work together to maintain balance in the system. Epigenetic reprogramming can occur with or without alterations or deletions to the existing DNA, potentially affecting chromatin. Methylation of DNA inhibits gene expression, while hydroxymethylation enhances gene expression. The first type of reprogramming involves cytosine at its fifth carbon in the pyrimidine ring, known as CpG islands. This can include methylation, hydroxymethylation, formylation, or carboxylation. The second method is histone modification, which can involve acetylation, methylation, phosphorylation, ubiquitination, or sumoylation. This reprogramming, which occurs in germ cells, has the ability to pass these changes on to

S. no.	Gene	Cytogenic location	Anomalies
1	*AR*	Xq12	X inactivation
2	*FSHR*	2p16.3	Gene variation
3	*FTO*	16q12.2	SNP rs9939609
4	*CAPN10*	2q37.3	Polymorphism
5	*CYPA1A*	15q24.1	T6235C
6	*CYP11A1*	15q24.1	SNP rs4077582
7	*CYP17A1*	10q24.32	T>C
8	*CYP1A1*	15q24.1	Ile/Val
9	*CYP21A2*	6p21.33	Heterozygous mutation
10	*CYP3A7*	7q22.1	Variant allele
11	*CYP19A1*	15q21.2	Arg264Cys

Table 1.
Genomic varients related to pcos.

offspring. Next-generation sequencing (NGS) is used to identify this genetic reprogramming. The various physiological processes related to follicular development, steroidogenesis, glucose metabolism, insulin regulation, and inflammatory mediation are associated with luteinising hormone/choriogonadotropin receptor (LHCGR), FST, LMNA, PPARGC1, and EPHX1 genes. In PCOS, there is decreased methylation and over-expression of LHCGR and PPAR-gamma genes. Obesity also plays an epigenetic modifier in the development of PCOS. These two epigenetic modifications complement each other, resulting in changes in DNA. Two hit theories include the first hit in intrauterine life, and the second one is a provocative factor after delivery in her lifetime. A genome-wide association study identifies a gene that regulates gonadotropin secretion, action, and ovarian function. These genes are FSHB (follicle-stimulating hormone B polypeptide), LHCGR (luteinising hormone/choriogonadotropin receptor), FSHR (follicle-stimulating hormone receptor), anti-Mullerian hormone (AMH), and DENND1A (DENN domain-containing 1A) and genes associated with metabolism, such as THADA (thyroid-adenoma-associated gene) and INSR (insulin receptor).

3. Environmental factors

Endocrine-disrupting chemicals (EDC) are present in whatever we use in our day-to-day life. These are phenols or halogens like chlorine and bromine [4]. They mimic steroid hormone action. Longer and uninterrupted exposure to EDCs from prenatal to adolescence is a causative factor of PCOS [5]. Bisphenol A (BPA), which is used for packaging food and drink and many other purposes, interferes with oogenesis [4, 6]. BPA acts on granulosa cells and reduces the expression of aromatase enzyme and the production of oestrogen, thereby interfering with oocyte development and maturation. BPA is also a potent ligand for sex hormone-binding globulin (SHBG) and replaces testosterone thereby increasing free testosterone concentration. High androgen deactivates the uridine diphosphate-glucuronosyl transferase enzyme and decreases BPA clearance in the liver. Thereby, it increases the concentration of free BPA in blood, leading to further negative effects on the ovaries [4, 6–8]. BPA upregulates adipogenesis-related genes and activates glucocorticoid receptors, thus acting as an obesogenic. BPA also gives rise to the release of interleukin 6 (IL6) and tumour necrosis factor α (TNF-α), which prompts adiposity and insulin resistance. BPA also affects glucose homeostasis by directly influencing pancreatic cells. Advanced glycation end products (AGEs), also called glycotoxins, are pro-inflammatory molecules affecting women's health. They interact with the surface receptor called RAGE (receptor for AGE) and stimulate proinflammatory pathways and oxidative stress [9, 10]. It prompts adiposeness. Increased body mass index decreases the clearance of glycotoxin and is responsible for its deposition in ovaries. This worsens the inflammatory process and metabolic syndrome of PCOS [9].

4. Physical and emotional stress

Chronic stress causes hypertrophy and hyperplasia of adipocytes, stimulating adipocrine secretion attraction and activation of stromal fat immune cells [11]. Chronic stress also causes increased levels of inflammatory cytokines, like IL-6 and TNF-α, and affects oxidant-antioxidant balance. It has a role in increased insulin resistance. Stress induces hypothalamic-pituitary axis to release cortisol. Cortisol leads to IR by stimulating visceral fat accumulation, gluconeogenesis, lipolysis, and increased glucose production in liver [12]. Stress effect on PCOS may refer to intervention with anti-Mullerian hormone (AMH) and changing sex hormone levels [12, 13]. Recent research studies on animals have shown that AMH stimulates LH release and increases the gonadotropin-releasing hormone, thereby linking AMH to endocrine instability.

Diet with saturated fatty acids (SFAs): it produces an inflammatory status [14] and lowers insulin sensitivity [15]. Vitamin D deficiency aggravates comorbidities associated with PCOS [15, 16]. Vitamin D deficiency increases insulin resistance by causing chronic inflammation [15, 17]. Vitamin D supplementation may have a beneficial effect on AMH and antral follicle count (AFC) in women with PCOS [18].

There is a decreased response of cells to insulin in women with PCOS. It is seen both in lean and obese PCOS women. Insufficient response to insulin is tissue-specific. Insulin response in ovarian tissue and adrenal is not affected [19, 20]. Insulin promotes growth of ovarian follicle and steroidogenesis. Insulin like growth factor coacts with LH. Hyperinsulinemia increases androgen production from ovary [21]. IR independently augment CYP17A1 activity, the secretory enzyme in androstenedione and testosterone production [22]. Hyperinsulinemia decreases hepatic SHBG and elevates free testosterone levels in blood. It also increases IGF-1 production in liver, which increases androgen production by stimulating theca cells. Hyperinsulinemia also stimulates LH receptors in pituitary and increases both frequency and amplitude of LH secretion. Insulin has been found to be associated with enhanced pituitary gonadotropin sensitivity to GnRH. Thus, hyperinsulinemia promotes GnRH neuron activity. It stimulates adiposeness and lipogenesis and inhibits lipolysis. Insulin resistance causes a decrease in omentin level that is independent of the patient's body mass index (BMI). Insulin's indirect effect on PCOS is enhanced by pituitary gonadotropin sensitivity to GnRH, and hyperinsulinemia promotes GnRH neuron activity [23]. Hyperglycaemia causes inflammation by secreting TNF-α from mononuclear cells (MNCs) [24].

5. Hyperandrogenism

It reduces sex hormone-binding globulin and increases serum-free testosterone. In women with PCOS, higher testosterone is converted to estrone in adipose tissue. Estrone is converted to estradiol, which affects follicular growth and alters LH and FSH ratio, which affects ovulation [10]. Hyperandrogenism upregulates AMH level, which inhibits follicular growth and ovulation. IGF-II level, which is positively related to follicular diameter, decreased in follicular fluid caused by increased androgen level. Hyperandrogenism increases LH level. Hyperandrogenism adds to PCOS-related inflammatory factors, insulin resistance, and oxidative stress. PCOS women have adipose tissue similar to men because of hyperandrogenism. Increased levels of white blood cell, C-reactive protein (CRP), and other inflammatory biomarkers in peripheral blood are associated with PCOS [25]. Inflammation induces hyperandrogenism. TNF-αexacerbates insulin resistance. IL-1 affects the FSH and LH receptors, which interfere with follicular development and ovulation.

6. Oxidative stress

It denotes an imbalance between pro-oxidants and antioxidants. Oxidative stress molecules include reactive oxygen species (ROS) (e.g., O^{2-}, H_2O_2, and OH^-) and reactive nitrogen species (RNS). Excess production of oxidative chemicals causes various damage to vital molecules such as lipids, proteins, and DNA. Oxidative stress inhibits the insulin signalling pathway and adds to IR. Oxidative stress leads to obesity [26].

7. Obesity

Obesity can lead to insulin resistance, hyperinsulinemia, and hyperandrogenism. Visceral obesity can cause an increase in non-esterified fatty acids (NEFAs) in the bloodstream. Skeletal muscles utilise NEFAs as an energy source instead of glucose. This can cause hyperglycaemia, triggering a rapid response in the pancreas and resulting in hyperinsulinemia. Visceral fat adipocytes undergo necrosis in response to catecholamines. This leads to release of cytokines like TNF and IL6, which are further responsible for adrenal steroidogenesis and hyperandrogenemia. This obesity-induced inflammatory process is also responsible for impairing insulin clearance, hence also contributing to hyperinsulinemia. Adipocytes produce high levels of leptin, which inhibits the expression of aromatase mRNA in granulosa cells and prevents the conversion of androgens to oestrogen and thus hampers ovarian folliculogenesis. Adiponectin, secreted by adipocytes, is insulin-sensitising, anti-diabetic, and has anti-inflammatory properties. Visceral fat secretes lower levels of adiponectin compared to subcutaneous fat. Omentin-1, a chemical secreted by adipose tissue, enhances IGF-1-induced progesterone and estradiol secretion, stimulates the expression of steroidogenic acute regulatory protein and CYP450 aromatase, and improves IGF-1 receptor signalling in adipose tissue. The accumulation of lipids in non-adipose tissues, known as lipotoxicity, can lead to oxidative/endoplasmic reticulum stress associated with inflammation and insulin resistance. Excessive fatty acids in muscles and liver can induce insulin resistance through serine phosphorylation of the insulin receptor by diacylglycerol.

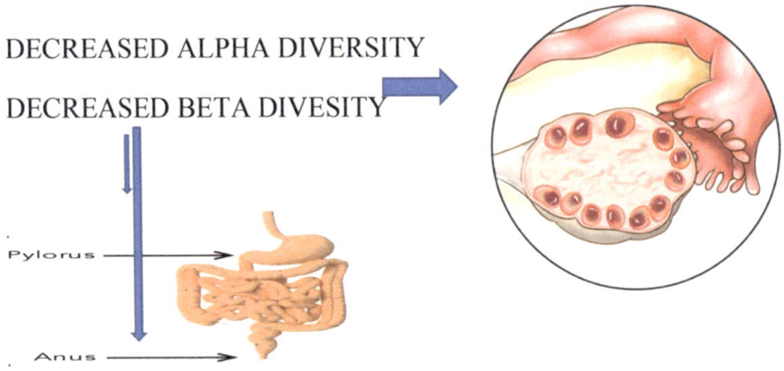

Figure 1.
Gut microbiome and PCOS.

8. Gut microbiome

The clinical manifestations of PCOS women are also associated with the brain-gut axis [27]. The release of endotoxin by the gut microbiome as a response to gut inflammation is found to be a contributing factor in PCOS. Various gut microbiota play a role in maintaining physiological balance and preserving structural integrity and histological homeostasis. Additionally, the gut microbiome is involved in the production of vitamins, short-chain free fatty acids, and conjugated linoleic acid. It also plays a role in the biotransformation of bile acids, ammonia synthesis, and detoxification. Short-chain fatty acids such as acetate, butyrate, and propionate are produced by the gut microbiome and have anti-inflammatory, anticarcinogenic, and immunomodulatory effects [28]. The metabolism of butyrate and propionate is important for energy metabolism, as it regulates the gluconeogenesis process and cholesterol metabolism. Furthermore, the gut microbiome modulates the immune system [29]. The diversity of the microbiome is crucial for restoring the host's health. Obese individuals with PCOS have lower alpha and beta diversity compared to those without PCOS [30]. The main species of firmicutes in the human gut are *Lactobacillus*, *Clostridium*, and *Ruminococcus*. Among these, *Lactobacillus* has a direct association with PCOS and its impact on human health [31]. Liu et al. observed a decrease in Ruminococcaceae and *Clostridium* in obese individuals with PCOS [32]. The presence of the Proteobacteria phylum, specifically *Salmonella*, is associated with PCOS. Bacteroidetes, on the other hand, were significantly lower in the stools of PCOS patients and were associated with reproductive hormones such as thyroid-stimulating hormone (TSH) and luteinising hormone (LH) [33]. There is an immune neurological network formed by the central nervous system, intestinal neural network, and pituitary adrenal axis. Correlation between gut microbiome and PCOS will lead to a newer management option for women suffering from PCOS (**Figure 1**).

9. Neuroendocrine correlation

Polycystic ovary syndrome is symbolised by excess androgen and ovulatory dysfunction. There is a rapid pulse frequency of gonadotrophin-releasing hormone due to the decreased sensitivity to the progesterone and oestrogen feedback inhibition at the level of hypothalamus [34]. The pulsatile release of GnRH is from the median

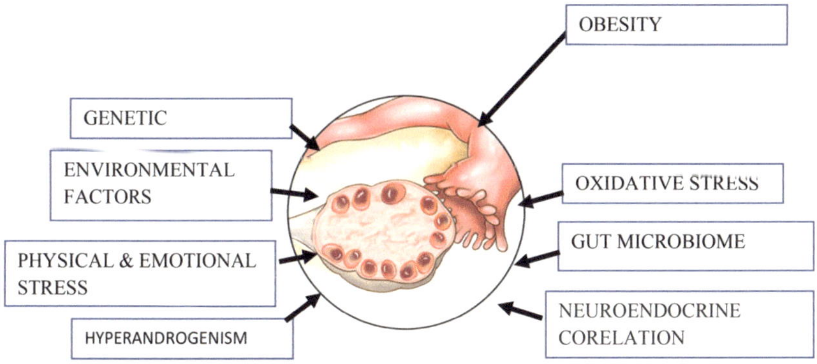

Figure 2.
Causes of PCOS.

eminence, which controls the pulsatile LH secretion from the anterior pituitary. This hormonal imbalance leads to increased LH and FSH ratio which accounts for excess androgen secretion from ovary and arrest of follicular growth and oligo ovulation [35]. The various neuronal modulators associated with PCOS are KDNy neurons, kisspeptin released from hypothalamus, γ-aminobutyric acid (GABA), AMH, and others. There is an increased level of kisspeptin in women with PCOS. Thus, the blending effect of kisspeptin and LH is lost in PCOS women, resulting in dysregulated gonadotrophin-releasing hormone pulsatility. γ-Aminobutyric acid (GABA) and anti-Mullerian hormone also stimulate gonadotrophin-releasing hormone neurons directly. GABA has an excitatory effect on gonadotrophin-releasing hormone neurons. Thus, an increased level of γ-aminobutyric acid (GABA) is found in cerebrospinal fluid in women with PCOS. Direct action of hyperandrogenism in brain might have a role in the development of PCOS traits [36]. Many clinical studies have found a positive correlation between PCOS and psychiatric disorders. A higher incidence of PCOS in bipolar disorder might be due to neurotransmitter imbalance on the neuroendocrine axis executing reproductive dysfunction [37]. Women suffering from depression have a 35% of occurrence of PCOS [38]. Studies show there is also an increased incidence of PCOS in women with epilepsy. Women using valproate have an increased incidence of PCOS due to increased GABA levels. A clinical trial has shown a favourable result by targeting KDNy neuron with Ank3 receptor antagonist in women with PCOS to decrease LH pulsatility [39]. Early response of antral follicle to dysregulated LH reaches the incipient end-stage resulting in ovarian morphology in women with PCOS (**Figure 2**).

10. Conclusion

The exact aetiology of PCOS is not known, and it may be multifactorial in origin. Genetic factors, metabolic factors, and environmental factors interplay in the pathophysiology of PCOS. Genomic studies have identified the various genes involved in gonadotropin secretion, gonadotropin action, ovarian follicular development, and insulin sensitivity. This genetic association, with their epigenetic regulators, are still under constant research, which will further improve the understanding of disease, thereby improving its diagnosis and treatment modalities. Newer research on neuroendocrine factors and gut microbiome will facilitate innovative approach for the management of PCOS and its consequences. Neuroendocrine and gut microbiome topics of research for the aetiology of PCOS are in early stage and mostly based on the mice model. Further research, specifically on humans, is required to establish these factors as the causative factors of PCOS, and that will open the innovative window for the management of this endocrine and metabolic disorder.

Author details

Subrat Panda[1*], Rituparna Das[2], Lisley Konar[1] and Manasi Singh[1]

1 AIIMS, Kalyani, India

2 AIIMS, Guwahati, India

*Address all correspondence to: pandadrsubrat@rediffmail.com

References

[1] Dunaif A. Insulin resistance and the polycystic ovary syndrome: Mechanism and implications for pathogenesis. Endocrine Reviews. 1997;**18**:774

[2] Goyal M, Dawood AS. Debates regarding lean patients with polycystic ovary syndrome: A narrative review. Journal of Human Reproductive Sciences. 2017;**10**:154

[3] Legro RS, Driscoll D, Strauss JF, Fox J, Dunaif A. Evidence for a genetic basis for hyperandrogenemia in polycystic ovary syndrome. Proceedings of the National Academy of Sciences. 1998;**95**:14956

[4] Rutkowska AZ, Diamanti-Kandarakis E. Polycystic ovary syndrome and environmental toxins. Fertility and Sterility. 2016;**106**(4):948-958. DOI: 10.1016/j.fertnstert.2016.08.031. Epub 2016 Aug 22

[5] Calina D, Docea AO, Golokhvast KS, Sifakis S, Tsatsakis A, Makrigiannakis A. Management of Endocrinopathies in pregnancy: A review of current evidence. International Journal of Environmental Research and Public Health. 2019;**16**(5):781. DOI: 10.3390/ijerph16050781

[6] Soave I, Occhiali T, Assorgi C, Marci R, Caserta D. Environmental toxin exposure in polycystic ovary syndrome women and possible ovarian neoplastic repercussion. Current Medical Research and Opinion. 2020;**36**(4):693-703. DOI: 10.1080/03007995.2020.1729108. Epub 2020 Feb 27

[7] Palioura E, Diamanti-Kandarakis E. Polycystic ovary syndrome (PCOS) and endocrine disrupting chemicals (EDCs). Reviews in Endocrine & Metabolic Disorders. 2015;**16**(4):365-371. DOI: 10.1007/s11154-016-9326-7

[8] Palioura E, Diamanti-Kandarakis E. Industrial endocrine disruptors and polycystic ovary syndrome. Journal of Endocrinological Investigation. 2013;**36**(11):1105-1111. DOI: 10.1007/BF03346762

[9] Botros N, Sluik D, van Waateringe RP, de Vries JHM, Geelen A, Feskens EJM. Advanced glycation end-products (AGEs) and associations with cardio-metabolic, lifestyle, and dietary factors in a general population: The NQplus study. Diabetes/Metabolism Research and Reviews. Jul 2017;**33**(5). DOI: 10.1002/dmrr.2892. Epub 2017 Apr 17. PMID: 28249105

[10] Li Y, Chen C, Ma Y, Xiao J, Luo G, Li Y, et al. Multi-system reproductive metabolic disorder: Significance for the pathogenesis and therapy of polycystic ovary syndrome (PCOS). Life Sciences. 2019;**228**:167-175. DOI: 10.1016/j.lfs.2019.04.046

[11] Stefanaki C, Pervanidou P, Boschiero D, Chrousos GP. Chronic stress and body composition disorders: Implications for health and disease. Hormones (Athens, Greece). 2018;**17**(1):33-43. DOI: 10.1007/s42000-018-0023-7. Epub 2018 Apr 27

[12] Steegers-Theunissen RPM, Wiegel RE, Jansen PW, Laven JSE, Sinclair KD. Polycystic ovary syndrome: A brain disorder characterized by eating problems originating during puberty and adolescence. International Journal of Molecular Sciences. 2020;**21**(21):8211. DOI: 10.3390/ijms21218211

[13] Yang S, Yang C, Pei R, Li C, Li X, Huang X, et al. Investigation on

the association of occupational stress with risk of polycystic ovary syndrome and mediating effects of HOMA-IR. Gynecological Endocrinology. 2018;**34**(11):961-964. DOI: 10.1080/09513590.2018.1460340. Epub 2018 Jul 25

[14] Szczuko M, Kikut J, Szczuko U, Szydłowska I, Nawrocka-Rutkowska J, Ziętek M, et al. Nutrition strategy and life style in polycystic ovary syndrome-narrative review. Nutrients. 2021;**13**(7):2452. DOI: 10.3390/nu13072452

[15] Faghfoori Z, Fazelian S, Shadnoush M, Goodarzi R. Nutritional management in women with polycystic ovary syndrome: A review study. Diabetes and Metabolic Syndrome: Clinical Research and Reviews. 2017;**11**(Suppl. 1):S429-S432. DOI: 10.1016/j.dsx.2017.03.030. Epub 2017 Apr 5

[16] Muscogiuri G, Altieri B, de Angelis C, Palomba S, Pivonello R, Colao A, et al. Shedding new light on female fertility: The role of vitamin D. Reviews in Endocrine & Metabolic Disorders. 2017;**18**(3):273-283. DOI: 10.1007/s11154-017-9407-2

[17] Ciebiera M, Esfandyari S, Siblini H, Prince L, Elkafas H, Wojtyła C, et al. Nutrition in Gynecological diseases: Current perspectives. Nutrients. 2021;**13**(4):1178. DOI: 10.3390/nu13041178

[18] Bacanakgil BH, İlhan G, Ohanoğlu K. Effects of vitamin D supplementation on ovarian reserve markers in infertile women with diminished ovarian reserve. Medicine (Baltimore). 2022;**101**(6):e28796. DOI: 10.1097/MD.0000000000028796

[19] Dabadghao P. Polycystic ovary syndrome in adolescents. Best Practice & Research. Clinical Endocrinology & Metabolism. 2019;**33**(3):101272. DOI: 10.1016/j.beem.2019.04.006. Epub 2019 Apr 13

[20] Rothenberg SS, Beverley R, Barnard E, Baradaran-Shoraka M, Sanfilippo JS. Polycystic ovary syndrome in adolescents. Best Practice & Research. Clinical Obstetrics & Gynaecology. 2018;**48**:103-114. DOI: 10.1016/j.bpobgyn.2017.08.008. Epub 2017 Sep 1

[21] Rosenfield RL, Ehrmann DA. The pathogenesis of polycystic ovary syndrome (PCOS): The hypothesis of PCOS as functional ovarian Hyperandrogenism revisited. Endocrine Reviews. 2016;**37**(5):467-520. DOI: 10.1210/er.2015-1104. Epub 2016 Jul 26

[22] Zeng X, Xie YJ, Liu YT, Long SL, Mo ZC. Polycystic ovarian syndrome: Correlation between hyperandrogenism, insulin resistance and obesity. Clinica Chimica Acta. 2020;**502**:214-221. DOI: 10.1016/j.cca.2019.11.003. Epub 2019 Nov 13

[23] Baskind NE, Balen AH. Hypothalamic-pituitary, ovarian and adrenal contributions to polycystic ovary syndrome. Best Practice & Research. Clinical Obstetrics & Gynaecology. 2016;**37**:80-97. DOI: 10.1016/j.bpobgyn.2016.03.005. Epub 2016 Apr 1

[24] Bannigida DM, Nayak BS, Vijayaraghavan R. Insulin resistance and oxidative marker in women with PCOS. Archives of Physiology and Biochemistry. 2020;**126**(2):183-186. DOI: 10.1080/13813455.2018.1499120. Epub 2018 Nov 17

[25] Rudnicka E, Suchta K, Grymowicz M, Calik-Ksepka A, Smolarczyk K, Duszewska AM, et al. Chronic low grade inflammation in

pathogenesis of PCOS. International Journal of Molecular Sciences. 2021;**22**(7):3789. DOI: 10.3390/ijms22073789

[26] Mancini A, Bruno C, Vergani E, d'Abate C, Giacchi E, Silvestrini A. Oxidative stress and low-grade inflammation in polycystic ovary syndrome: Controversies and new insights. International Journal of Molecular Sciences. 2021;**22**(4):1667. DOI: 10.3390/ijms22041667

[27] Gu Y, Zhou G, Zhou F, Li Y, Wu Q, He H, et al. Gut and vaginal microbiomes in PCOS: Implications for Women's health. Frontiers in Endocrinology (Lausanne). 2022;**13**:808508. DOI: 10.3389/fendo.2022.808508

[28] Chambers ES, Byrne CS, Morrison DJ, Murphy KG, Preston T, Tedford C, et al. Dietary supplementation with inulin-propionate ester or inulin improves insulin sensitivity in adults with overweight and obesity with distinct effects on the gut microbiota, plasma metabolome and systemic inflammatory responses: A randomised cross-over trial. Gut. 2019;**68**(8):1430-1438. DOI: 10.1136/gutjnl-2019-318424. Epub 2019 Apr 10

[29] Belkaid Y, Harrison OJ. Homeostatic immunity and the microbiota. Immunity. 2017;**46**(4):562-576. DOI: 10.1016/j.immuni.2017.04.008

[30] Kho ZY, Lal SK. The human gut microbiome–A potential controller of wellness and disease. Frontiers in Microbiology. 2018;**9**:1835

[31] Rinninella E, Raoul P, Cintoni M, Franceschi F, Miggiano GA, Gasbarrini A, et al. What is the healthy gut microbiota composition? A changing ecosystem across age, environment, diet, and diseases. Microorganisms. 2019;**7**(1):14

[32] Liu R, Zhang C, Shi Y, Zhang F, Li L, Wang X, et al. Dysbiosis of gut microbiota associated with clinical parameters in polycystic ovary syndrome. Frontiers in Microbiology. 2017;**8**:324

[33] Lindheim L, Bashir M, Münzker J, Trummer C, Zachhuber V, Leber B, et al. Alterations in gut microbiome composition and barrier function are associated with reproductive and metabolic defects in women with polycystic ovary syndrome (PCOS): A pilot study. PLoS One. 2017;**12**(1):e0168390. DOI: 10.1371/journal.pone.0168390

[34] Garg A, Patel B, Abbara A, et al. Treatments targeting neuroendocrine dysfunction in polycystic ovary syndrome (PCOS). Clinical Endocrinology. 2022;**97**:156-164. DOI: 10.1111/cen.14704

[35] Katulski K, Podfigurna A, Czyzyk A, et al. Kisspeptin and LH pulsatile temporal coupling in PCOS patients. Endocrine. 2018;**61**:149-157. DOI: 10.1007/s12020-018-1609-1

[36] Caldwell AS, Edwards MC, Desai R, Jimenez M, Gilchrist RB, Handelsman DJ, et al. Neuroendocrine androgen action is a key extraovarian mediator in the development of polycystic ovary syndrome. National Academy of Sciences of the United States of America. 2017;**114**(16):E3334-E3343

[37] Qadri S, Hussain A, Bhat MH, Baba AA. Polycystic ovary syndrome in bipolar affective disorder: A hospital-based study. Indian Journal of Psychological Medicine. 2018;**40**(2):121-128. DOI: 10.4103/IJPSYM.IJPSYM_284_17

[38] Sadeghi HM, Adeli I, Calina D, Docea AO, Mousavi T, Daniali M, et al.

Polycystic ovary syndrome: A comprehensive review of pathogenesis, management, and drug repurposing. International Journal of Molecular Sciences. 6 Jan 2022;**23**(2):583. DOI: 10.3390/ijms23020583. PMID: 35054768; PMCID: PMC8775814

[39] George JT, Kakkar R, Marshall J, Scott ML, Finkelman RD, Ho TW, et al. Neurokinin b receptor antagonism in women with polycystic ovary syndrome: A randomized, placebo-controlled trial. The Journal of Clinical Endocrinology and Metabolism. 2016;**101**:4313-4432

Chapter 4

Would Non-coding RNA Resolve the Polycystic Ovary Syndrome (PCOS) Puzzle?

Rana Alhamdan

Abstract

Polycystic ovary syndrome (PCOS) is the most common endocrine heterogeneous reproductive disorder. This metabolic disease affects around 5–10% of women and accounts for 75% of anovulatory infertility all over the world. The complexity of the disease as manifested by the involvement of multiple underlying mechanisms and the lack of specific and sensitive biomarkers, make it difficult to timely manage and treat the disease. Remarkably, genetic, epigenetics, and environmental variations may contribute considerably to the pathogenicity of PCOS. Recent investigations indicated that non-coding RNAs (ncRNA) were involved in the occurrence and development of PCOS. Thus, this chapter aimed to summarize the current knowledge around the expression and dysregulation of ncRNA in human PCOS.

Keywords: polycystic ovarian syndrome (PCOS), infertility, non-coding RNA (ncRNA), micro RNAs (miRNAs), Long non-coding RNAs (lncRNAs)

1. Introduction

PCOS is the most common endocrine heterogeneous reproductive disorder. This metabolic disease affects around 5–10% of women and accounts for 75% of anovulatory infertility all over the world [1]. The fundamental features of this condition are oligo- or anovulation, hyperandrogenism, and polycystic ovaries. Women with PCOS may also develop other disorders, including type II diabetes, obesity, dyslipidemia, endometrial cancer, and insulin resistance (IR), in addition to being at risk of cardiovascular diseases [2]. Considering the complexity and diversity of this disorder, a deeper thinking and wider study of its etiology is certainly needed. In clinical settings, diagnosis is mainly based on the presentation of no less than two out of the three Rotterdam agreed main symptoms. These include polycystic ovaries, irregular periods, and high androgens. Therefore, the expert diagnostic opinion is now based on pelvic ultrasound examination and hormonal blood tests. This can emphasize the growing need for a specific and sensitive biomarker for the diagnosis of this condition [3].

Over the past two decades, a striking finding has indicated the presence of large amounts of non-protein-coding sequences in the genome of complex organisms [4, 5]. These previously named ‘transcriptional noise” sequences have now been shown to play multiple crucial biological roles and are referred to as non-coding RNAs (ncRNA). The involvement of those ncRNAs in the occurrence and development of PCOS has recently been indicated. A differential significant expression of ncRNAs has been found in the granulosa cells (GCs), follicular fluid (FF), Theca cells (TCs), serum, and plasma of patients with PCOS when compared to non-PCOS women [6, 7]. Therefore, this chapter aimed to provide an updated narrative review summarizing the current knowledge around the presence and dysregulated expression of ncRNAs. The chapter will review two main ncRNA regulators (microRNA (miRNAs), and long ncRNAs (lncRNAs)) and frame the discussion in the context of linking ncRNAs to the pathogenicity of PCOS as well as the possibility of using them as a biomarker to resolve the puzzle of PCOS.

1.1 Overview of ncRNAs

A significant amount of the human genome encodes functional transcripts that are destined for translation into proteins. Only recently, new classes of ncRNAs have been identified and were classified by length into small ncRNAs (sncRNAs) transcripts of small RNA sequences of <200 nucleotides and transcripts >200 nucleotides that lack any defined open frames and called lncRNA [5, 8, 9]. sncRNAs are further classified into miRNAs, small interfering RNA (siRNA), piwi-interacting RNA (piRNA), and transfer RNA (tRNA), small nuclear RNA (snRNA) [8]. Advanced sequencing technology led to the discovery of some of the underlying molecular mechanisms linking those ncRNAs with PCOS. It highlighted some precise and feasible biomarkers, of which miRNA and lncRNA have been the most well-characterized as functional ncRNAs in PCOS [5, 9, 10].

1.1.1 miRNAs and lncRNAs

ncRNAs are key regulators of gene expression and chromatin structures. They have particularly been shown to be relevant since the early stages of germline development.

miRNAs are small single-strand RNAs (22–23 nucleotide (nt) long). It plays a crucial biological role in regulating protein expression via either gene degradation or silencing. It acts as a core element to mediate gene and protein interactions at a multiple intra- and inter-cellular site to regulate their functions [11]. Hence, they are heavily available in biological fluids, a feature that facilitates their use as a biomarker research target.

Their biosynthesis is orchestrated at multiple events by which miRNAs are transcribed in the nucleus into a large primary form (pri-miRNAs). The immature pri-miRNAs are then methylated and subsequently processed by the DORSHA-DGCR8 complex and transferred to the cytoplasm. The cytoplasm is where pri-miRNAs are cleaved by DICER to form the mature double-stranded miRNA (22 nt), which are incorporated into a ribonuclear vesicle and form the RNA-induced silencing complex (RISC) [8, 11, 12].

lncRNAs, on the other hand, are typically longer than 200 nt. They are abundantly generated from 80–90% non-coding modulatory elements in the human genome and account for 60,000 lncRNA. Functional studies have recently classified the molecular mechanisms of lncRNAs into four types: guide, signal, decoy, and scaffold. They possess their regulatory role at the transcriptional, post-transcriptional processing levels, chromatin modification, and epigenetic modulation. Like miRNAs, they are radially available in body fluids and present in exosomes. A fact that makes them a good candidate as a non-invasive biomarker research tool.

LncRNAs, like other ncRNA, exhibit a complex three-dimensional structure and share a similar biosynthesis pathway. Based on their positional properties, they can be easily transcribed by polymerase II, polyadenylated, and spliced from different genomic sites. Owing to this property, lncRNAs are grouped into (1) natural antisense transcripts, (2) stand-alone, (3) pseudogenes, (4) intronic transcripts, and (5) enhancer RNA, promotor-associated, and divergent transcripts. LncRNAs lack open reading frames (PRFs); however, they exhibit a high tendency for cell-specific expression and possess a 3-terminal process specificity.

Both miRNAs and lncRNAs are present in abundance in body fluids and various cell types, and they have become a hot research topic for investigations related to PCOS diagnostic and therapeutic biomarker targets.

2. ncRNA and PCOS

To explore the cause, we need to critically assess the problem. This will lead us to explore the available knowledge associated with this disorder and further link that to how ncRNAs may contribute to the physiology and pathophysiology of PCOS.

Gonadotropin-releasing hormone (GnRH) is typically high in PCOS, leading to increased secretion of pituitary luteinizing hormone (LH). Consequently, ovarian androgen levels increase, leading to lower follicle-stimulating hormone (FSH) production by the pituitary gland. This would result in egg maturation issues and, therefore, anovulation. Moreover, numerous small follicles are observed in the ovary. In addition, altered steroidogenesis will result in abnormal production of estrogen (E2), progesterone (P4), and androgens [9]. Insulin resistance (IR) has also been described as a momentous cause of PCOS [6].

A vast number of ncRNAs have been observed altered in various reproductive tissues and body fluids from PCOS women. Their aberrant expression has been associated with abnormal ovarian cell apoptosis and/or proliferation, steroidogenesis, IRs, as well as adipocyte dysfunction among PCOS patients compared to healthy controls.

2.1 The role of ncRNAs in PCOS-associated ovarian steroidogenesis

Androgen production is vital for estrogen synthesis. Thus, the malfunction and/or incomplete conversion of androgens to estrogens cause hyperandrogenism (HA). PCOS is characterized by the dysregulation and increased production of the six main androgens: free testosterone (fT), testosterone (TT), androstenedione (A), sex hormone binding globulin (SHBG), 17-hydroxy progesterone (17-OHP), and dehydroepiandrosterone sulfate (DHEA [13]). Hyperandrogenism is substantially attributed to the ovaries and adrenals and with minimal contribution from fatty tissues. The imbalance in these hormones negatively impacts follicle development and oocyte maturation, leading to infertility. The etiologies associated with androgen excess are not solely uncovered and are still controversial. One possible reason is the increased P450 steroidogenic enzymatic activity, and another might be androgen receptor (AR) malfunction, cortisol metabolism defects, and/or the overproduction of androgen by TCs in response to LH overstimulation [14, 15]. It has been suggested that increased testosterone bioavailability in women with PCOS is the result of decreased SHBG [14].

AR has been proposed implicated and was reported to be highly expressed in patients with PCOS [16]. A growing body of evidence has indicated a regulatory role of ncRNAs in the sex steroids-associated physiological mechanisms [17].

2.1.1 miRNAs

The statistical significance of several **miRNAs** has already been documented as clinical biomarkers for PCOS [7, 18]. However, the complexity of the mechanisms involved in sex hormone production makes it harder to define those guilty miRNAs. A positive relationship has been indicated between miR-592 and LH/chorionic gonadotropin receptor (LH/CGH), a vital element in the HA-PCOS-involved mechanism [19]. In PCOS women, LH overstimulation has been shown to stimulate the expression of Pak3, thus down-regulating miR-125b-5p expression and leading to ERK1/2 signaling trigger, consequently, the increase expression of androgen synthesis-related enzymes and testosterone production [20]. The dysregulation of miR-23a and miR-146a has been found to inversely correlate with the significance of PCOS development. Both miRNAs were identified as negative regulators of serum testosterone [21, 22]. The overexpression of miR-278 and miR-181a has been shown to negatively regulate aromatase activity, thus leading to lower estrogen synthesis [23, 24]. Adding to those players modulating steroid synthesis, miR-34C, miR-9, miR-135a, miR-18b, and miR-32 have been found implicated [25]. miR-96-5P has also been shown to modulate E2 synthesis via the inhibition of serum, FF, and/or GC forkhead transcription factor (FOXO1) expression and its downstream genes [26]. miR-200b has also been proposed as a downstream target for AR via the hypothalamic-pituitary-ovarian axis (HPO-A) and may act as an actress in the processes leading to HA-PCOS [27]. Moreover, miR-320 is a controversial miRNA that has been once reported to be upregulated and next to be downregulated. The first group studied the expression of miR-320 in the FF of PCOS. They suggested the involvement of this miRNA in the inhibition of E2F1/SF1 proteins, thus leading to the downregulation of estradiol release into the FF [28]. However, the second study reported a significantly lower expression of miR-320 in PCOS when compared to controls and proposed a role of this miRNA in regulating steroidogenesis [29]. Despite the discrepancies between the studies, which might be due to the differences in the experimental settings and patients' population, miR-320 appears to have a direct relevance to the HA-PCOS phenotype.

It has been suggested that miRNA-423-3P may act guilty for the dysregulation of progesterone production by the TCs. A significant reduction of AdipoR2 (adiponectin receptor 2), a receptor to adiponectin, has been found in the TCs of women with PCOS. AdipoR2 has been shown to directly interact with miRNA-423-3P and thus may play an important role in the pathogenesis of PCOS [7].

2.1.2 lncRNAs

LncRNAs have been implicated in divergent indications of PCOS via various interaction networks including miRNAs and ceRNAs [10]. Chen et al. suggested that the lncRNA H19 can modulate steroidogenesis at the post-transcriptional levels. The group utilized an animal and a human model to demonstrate that H19 disturbance may alter androgen production via a Cyp17-related mechanism and can be an important player in the pathogenicity of PCOS-associated HA [17]. Another group demonstrated an inhibitory effect of lncRNA HUPCOS on CYP11 activity through the interaction with RNA-binding protein with multiple splicing (RBPMS). Via which, this lncRNA was positively correlated to FF testosterone in PCOS individuals [30]. Similarly, lncRNA OC1 silencing experiments have indicated the role of this lncRNA to suppress aromatase activity in the GCs of women with PCOS [31]. Furthermore, lncRNA terminal binding protein 1 anti-sense (CTBP1-AS) is thought to be an important modulator of AR and can tightly correspond to TT [10]. Moreover, lncRNA Neat1 has been previously described as implicated in the regulation of follicle development and P4 function. LncRNA Neat1 knockout (KO) mice exhibited low serum P4 expression levels and CL malfunction and, thus, pregnancy failure [7]. Interestingly, lncRNA zinc finger anti-sense 1 (ZFAS1), exhibiting a chromosome 20q13 location, was found to play a role in stimulating the secretion of E2 and P4 in the GCs of PCOS women. This study explored the mechanistic network between lncRNA ZFAS1/miR-129/and high-mobility group box protein 1(HMGB1) in PCOS. Their work demonstrated that both ZFAS1 and HMGB1 were upregulated and miR-129 was downregulated in the GCs of PCOS patients and that the silencing or reversing the action of either may repress the endocrine disturbance leading to this pathological condition [32].

These insights can indicate the complex interaction network between both miRNAs and lncRNAs to modulate the endocrine disturbance associated with the PCOS phenotype. Thus, further work is required to highlight the possible use of these ncRNAs as a potential therapeutic target. A summary of miRNAs and lncRNAs included in this section is provided in **Table 1**.

miRNAs	lncRNAs	Findings	Reference
miR-592		Expression passively associated with LH/chorionic gonadotropin receptor (LH/CGH)	[19]
miR-125b-5p		Increase expression of androgen synthesis-related enzymes and testosterone production	[20]
miR-23a, miR-146a		Negative regulators of serum testosterone	[21, 22]
miR-278, miR-181a		Negatively regulate aromatase activity, leading to lower estrogen synthesis	[23, 24]
miR-34C, miR-9, miR-135a, miR-18b, and miR-32		Modulating steroid synthesis	[25]
miR-96-5P		Modulate E2 synthesis	[26]
miR-200b		Modulate E2 synthesis	[27]
miR-320		Regulating steroidogenesis	[28, 29]
miRNA-423-3P		Dysregulation of progesterone production	[7]
	lncRNA H19	Modulate steroidogenesis	[17]
	lncRNA HUPCOS	Positively correlated to FF testosterone in PCOS individuals	[30]
	lncRNA OC1	Suppress aromatase activity in the GCs	[31]
	CTBP1-AS	Modulator of AR and can correspond to TT	[10]
	lncRNA Neat1	Regulation of follicle development and P4 function	[7]
	ZFAS1	Endocrine disturbance via sponging miR-129	[32]

Table 1.
The role of ncRNAs in PCOS-associated ovarian steroidogenesis.

2.2 The role of ncRNAs in PCOS-associated IR

It sounds like there is a strong link between IR, HA, and PCOS-related infertility. IR in PCOS is caused by impaired insulin action and is marked by compensatory hyperinsulinemia (HI) and reduced insulin response to glucose overload [33]. It is because insulin plays a significant role in facilitating androgen secretion from the pituitary, ovaries, liver, and adrenal glands, and it acts as a co-gonadotropin to regulate ovarian steroidogenesis. Additionally, it can arrest ovarian follicular development, modulate LH pulsatility, and negatively regulate SHBG production [34]. Androgen excess can lead to a chain reaction with IR and HI. It is prevalent in 65–95% of women diagnosed with PCOS, and it has been found that obesity can exacerbate these conditions. IR can stimulate an increase in CYP17 enzymatic activity, which in turn inhibits SHBG levels, leading to increased serum fT levels [8, 14]. Interesting to note that HA in the ovaries can be attributed to the insulin growth factor-1 (ICF-1) receptor, which can play a role in mediating LH-induced TCs androgen overproduction [35].

2.2.1 miRNAs

IGF-1 signaling pathway in synergy with peroxidase proliferator receptor (PPAR) and angiopoietin, has been shown to contribute to PCOS. Interestingly, miR-223 has been indicated to have the potential to modulate this pathway [36]. The expression miR-222 has been reported to positively correlate with serum insulin from patients with PCOS [21, 37]. It is apparent that miR-146 is an important factor in IR and is believed to have a significant role in its pathogenesis. The expression of miR-146 triggers a series of proinflammatory signals that activate nuclear factor kappa B (NFkB), leading to the upregulation of miR-146a, which in turn initiates negative feedback and regulates immune response. However, during hyperglycemia, this miRNA is downregulated despite NFkB activation and proinflammatory response [33, 38]. It is interesting to note that according to Sang et al. [29], miR-320 and miR-132 have been suggested to play a role in modulating IR. The author predicted that RABSB and HMGA2 are the target genes for miR-320 and miR-132, respectively, and that both gene expression are altered by reduced levels of these miRNAs in the FF of women with PCOS [29]. One of the reported miRNAs to be elevated in PCOS individuals is miR-93. The overexpression of this miRNA has been associated with IR and was shown to correspond strongly with GLUT4 receptor suppression in adipose tissues in women with PCOS [39]. It has been found that miR-133a-3p is highly expressed in patients with PCOS as compared to controls. This miRNA inhibits the PI3K/AKT (PKB) signaling pathway, which plays a crucial role in insulin action. The insulin receptor substrate-1 activates PI3K, which activates AKT, the main downstream protein. However, in PCOS, IR leads to inhibition of the PI3K/AKT signaling pathway. Nevertheless, the mechanism is not yet fully understood and requires further investigation [38].

Moreover, a recent investigation on glucagon-like peptide 1 agonist receptor agonist (GLP-1RA) and dipeptidyl peptidase-4 (DPP-4) inhibitors have shown a relationship with altered expression of miRNAs such as mIR-222, miR-221, miR-33, miR-155-5, miR-6763, miR-75-5p, miR-197, miR-1197-3p, and miR-6356, which may have an impact on insulin sensitivity and contribute to the management of symptoms related to PCOS by increasing glucose metabolism and transport [33, 40–42].

Furthermore, an antagonistic glycolytic regulatory activity has been observed to be exhibited by miR-155-5p and miR-143-2p in PCOS-related follicular dysplasia [43]. miR-29, miR-19a, miR-1, and miR126 have also been suggested to modulate glucose uptake via PI3K signaling pathways [44].

2.2.2 lncRNAs

The role of **lncRNAs** in association with IR has been addressed in a few studies. Intriguingly, around 20 lncRNA were found to co-expressed with the neuropeptide Y1 receptor (NPY1R), a candidate gene for type 2 diabetes mellitus, and these co-expressed lncRNAs may have a significant role in the development of PCOS [5]. According to a study by Zhao et al. [34], using WGCNA analysis, six hub lncRNAs (RP11-151A6.4, LNC00475, RP11-54A4.2, TTTY14, RP1-93H18.1, and RP3-439F8.1) were found to be significantly associated with IRs in patients with PCOS. Of all six lncRNAs, lncRNA RP11-151A6.4 was identified to express at a significantly higher level in both subcutaneous and omental adipose tissues of patients with IR compared to healthy controls. Moreover, the expression levels of RP11-151A6.4 in ovarian GCs were increased in patients with PCOS compared to control patients with HI. These findings may suggest a significant role of this lncRNA in IR-related PCOS [34]. A limited number of studies have explored the relationship between lncRNAs and PCOS with IRs. However, the model used by Zhao and his colleagues, and the potential molecular candidates explored by the group could be crucial for future investigations and may help to understand the mechanisms of IRs. Thus, further investigation is urged to explore the possible pathogenic role of miRNAs and lncRNAs in patients with PCOS and IRs. A summary of miRNAs and lncRNAs included in this section is provided in **Table 2**.

2.3 The role of ncRNAs in PCOS-associated GCs proliferation and apoptosis

GCs play a crucial role in the growth and maturation of oocytes, and any dysfunction in these cells can contribute to abnormal folliculogenesis and hormone production. Thus, aberrant GC proliferation and apoptosis are believed to be a significant factor in the development of PCOS.

2.3.1 miRNAs

Several studies have profiled ncRNAs in GCs taken from women with and without PCOS. It has been shown that women with PCOS tend to have lower levels of miR-145 in their GCs. Interestingly, the upregulation of this miRNA not only inhibited cell proliferation but also promoted cell apoptosis in human GCs. Further investigations demonstrated that miR-145 can suppress the activation of the MAPK/ERK signaling pathway via binding to insulin receptor substrate 1(IRS1). Based on these findings, the author suggested that the inhibition of miR-145 levels may promote GC proliferation via IRS1/MAPK/ERK regulatory network in women with PCOS [45]. Mao et al. [46] have also reported lower expression of miR-29a-5p, 92b, and miR-126-5p in GCs of PCOS women, which could induce GC apoptosis [46]. The role of miR-486-5p, miR-3940-5p, miR-182, miR-206, miR-15a, and miR-204 in modulating ovarian GC proliferation and apoptosis have been reported. While miR-3940-5p was found to be upregulated, low expression of miR-182, miR-15a, miR-486-5p, miR-206, and

miRNAs	lncRNAs	Findings	References
miR-223		Modulate IGF-1 signaling pathway in synergy with PPAR and angiopoietin	[36]
miR-222		Positively correlate with serum insulin	[21, 37]
miR-146, miR-146a		Triggers a series of proinflammatory signals leading to the Initialization of negative feedback and regulates immune response	[33, 38]
miR-320, miR-132		Modulating IR	[29]
miR-93		Modulating IR	[39]
miR-133a-3p		Modulating IR	[38]
mIR-222, m*i*R-221, m*i*R-33, m*i*R-155-5, m*i*R-6763, *miR*-75-5p, m*i*R-197, m*i*R-1197-3p, and m*i*R-6356,		Increasing glucose metabolism and transport, associated with PCOS-related follicular dysplasia	[40, 41, 42]
miR-155-5p and miR-143-2p		Antagonistic glycolytic regulatory activity	[43]
miR-29, miR-19a, miR-1, and miR126		Modulate glucose uptake via PI3K signaling pathways	[44]
	lncRNAs (RP11-151A6.4, LNC00475, RP11-54A4.2, TTTY14, RP1-93H18.1, and RP3-439F8.1)	Their expression was significantly associated with IRs	[34]

Table 2.
The role of ncRNAs in PCOS-associated IR.

miR-204 has been observed in the GC of PCOS individuals when compared to healthy controls [14, 47, 48]. However, the profile of miR-486-5 in PCOS has been reported with contradicting results [49, 50].

It is well established that GCs are the primary site of endocrine signaling and estrogen synthesis in the ovaries. Thus, it is expected that the dysregulation of miRNAs in GC may contribute to the dearth of E2, a major feature of PCOS. Zhang et al. [51] reported a low expression of miR-320a in the CCs in females with PCOS when compared to healthy controls. The group proposed that miR-320a induced E2 deficiency via 320a/RUNX2/CYP11A1 (CYP19A1) regulatory pathway [51].

The overexpression of miR-93 has been reported in the GCs of PCOS patients. Jiang et al., further indicated that cdkn1a is the target gene of this miRNA and that the absence of this gene supported the stimulating proliferation role of miR-93, whereas the reintroduction of cdkn1a reversed this effect [52]. He et al. [53] have suggested that miR-141 and miR-200 expression in the GC of PCOS patients may target the PI3K/Wnt signaling pathway to inhibit their proliferation [53]. The significant upregulation of miR-513b, miR-509-3p, and miR-423-3p has been reported by several studies in the CCs of women with PCOS [50, 54, 55].

2.3.2 lncRNAs

It is interesting to note that Huang et al. [54] demonstrated that there was a significant upregulation of the expression of 620 **lncRNAs** in PCOS cumulus cells, with only three lncRNAs being downregulated [54]. Similarly, Liu et al. [55, 56] observed that 692 lncRNAs were upregulated and 170 lncRNAs were downregulated in PCOS GCs [56]. Chen et al., discovered that lncRNA hcp5 may play a role in promoting cell proliferation and apoptosis via the miR-27a-3p/IGF-1 axis in the human KGN cell line model [57]. Utilizing a knockout model, the Zhu group has demonstrated that ZFAS1 can potentially increase GC proliferation and inhibit apoptosis in PCOS [32]. Moreover, LINC00477 has been recently reported to be significantly highly expressed in PCOS women, and it is postulated that may promote PCOS by inhibiting the GCs proliferation and increasing apoptosis through sponging miR-128. The study demonstrated that the expression levels of this lncRNA in the serum can be used to distinguish PCOS individuals from healthy counterparts [58]. Furthermore, another study found that the lncRNA PVT1/miR-17-5p/PTEN axis may have a role in regulating E2

miRNAs	lncRNAs	Findings	Reference
miR-145		Inhibited GCs proliferation and promoted cell apoptosis	[45]
miR-29a-5p, 92b, and miR-126-5p		Induce GC apoptosis	[46]
miR-182, miR-15a, miR-486-5p, miR-206, and miR-204, miR-3940-5p		Modulating ovarian GC proliferation and apoptosis	[14, 47, 48]
miR-320a		Induced E2 deficiency	[51]
miR-93		Modulating ovarian GC proliferation and apoptosis	[52]
miR-141 and miR-200		Target the PI3K/Wnt signaling pathway to inhibit GCs proliferation	[53]
miR-513b, miR-509-3p, and miR-423-3p		Modulating ovarian GC proliferation and apoptosis	[50, 54, 55]
	lncRNA hcp5	Promoting GCs proliferation and apoptosis via the miR-27a-3p/IGF-1 axis	[57]
	ZFAS1	Increase GCs proliferation and inhibit apoptosis	[32].
	LINC00477	Inhibiting the GCs proliferation and increasing apoptosis through sponging miR-128	[58]
	lncRNA PVT1	Regulate GCs proliferation and apoptosis	[58]
	TUG1	Modulate GCs proliferation, aromatase expression and E2 biosynthesis in GCs	[59]
	HCG26	Modulating GC proliferation and steroidogenesis	[60]

Table 3.
The role of ncRNAs in PCOS-associated GCs proliferation and apoptosis.

and P4 secretion, as well as GC proliferation and apoptosis in PCOS [58]. It is interesting to note that Taurine upregulated 1 (TUG1) was found to be highly expressed in PCOS GCs and that was directly correlated to an increased AFC. Furthermore, TUG1 was primarily localized in the nuclei of human GCs. The findings that TUG1 silencing inhibited cell proliferation and regulated apoptosis and autophagy in MAPKs pathway-dependent and P21-dependent manners are also noteworthy. Moreover, the TUG1 knockdown model increased aromatase expression and E2 biosynthesis in GCs [59]. The results of a recent independent microarray analysis performed by Liu et al. [60] have demonstrated an increased expression of lncRNA human leukocyte antigen complex group 26 (HCG26) in PCOS patients when compared to their matched controls. Further functional analysis revealed that the knockdown of HCG26 inhibits cell proliferation while promoting aromatase gene expression and E2 production. These findings suggest that HCG26 plays a role in GC proliferation and steroidogenesis and thus contributes to the pathogenicity of PCOS [60]. On the whole, these data indicate the presence of different profiles of miRNAs and lncRNAs in GCs in individuals with PCOS compared to healthy controls. These ncRNAs (**Table 3**) may play various roles in cellular proliferation and apoptosis, hormone regulation, and angiogenesis.

3. Did ncRNA resolve the puzzle for PCOS?

Efforts to gain a better understanding of the molecular endogenous RNA networks affecting PCOS are vast. These studies successfully shed some light on the complicated interactions and functions in association with the endocrine and female reproductive system overall. The research demonstrated the crucial role of ncRNAs in forming a mutual functional endogenous network that can significantly develop and modulate a disease state.

Sequencing technology and transcriptomics analysis have been used by various groups to investigate potential ncRNAs as biomarkers for PCOS with varying biological significance. However, to agree on the statistical significance of any of the found biomarkers, it is important to take into consideration several factors. Among the most important are the p-value, the specificity and sensitivity of the fold change in PCOS and related symptoms, and how relevant the indicated role of the biomarker is [3]. The data available to date is contradictory, and very few ncRNAs can be defined as significant to the condition of PCOS. The reason for that can be related to the various types of samples and methods used by the different groups. Adding to the complexity of testing is the fact that PCOS is a multi-organ disorder, which means it can be affected by the various ncRNAs expressed in association with extracellular signaling. Therefore, it is important to study these functional biomolecules by utilizing more experimental investigations and large data build-up and analysis. Several models have been shown to be useful, such as the bioinformatics approach used by Zeng et al. The group was able to develop an RNA-drug network based on differentially expressed miRNAs and lncRNAs. This approach allows for the identification of molecular correlations among drugs and can guide future work in locating the underlying mechanisms and functional roles of these biomolecules in PCOS [3, 61]. Furthermore, studies on human cell lines such as KGN cells can also be promising, especially in studying intracellular signaling networks [60, 62]. This approach in combination with tissue and cell analysis is prominent to investigate biomolecular interactions and molecular mechanisms involved in follicular development and PCOS. Gene Ontology (GO) and pathway analysis with the Kyoto Encyclopedia of Genes and

Genomes (KEGG) has been used by several groups to discover significant correlations between ncRNAs biomarkers for PCOS in association with functional biological significance [3, 5]. The statistical significance and true causation analysis to point and define effective biomarkers for the diagnosis and treatment of PCOS require further clarity of the underlying mechanisms. Thus, the combination of these approaches mentioned above would be a good way to move forward in discovering the PCOS-associated therapeutic complexes.

4. Conclusion

In conclusion, PCOS is a condition associated with hormonal imbalances manifesting into infertility and other serious long-term health problems. Early and accurate diagnosis is crucial, as it can help prevent complications like diabetes. The fact that PCOS affects endocrine cellular functions is certainly concerning and urges more work to clearly define the accurate causation of the condition. The advancement in sequencing technology is promising and can help us expect reliable ncRNA biomarkers that can be used in clinical settings worldwide soon. Further research is needed to explore complex networks of ncRNAs/RNAs and protein combinations and useful functional signaling pathways. This could help unveil and resolve the PCOS puzzle.

Conflict of interest

The authors declare no conflict of interest.

Author details

Rana Alhamdan
King Faisal Specialist Hospital and Research Center, Riyadh, Saudi Arabia

*Address all correspondence to: amsf199705@hotmail.co.uk

References

[1] Asunción M, Calvo RM, San Millán JL, Sancho J, Avila S, Escobar-Morreale HCF. A prospective study of the prevalence of the polycystic ovary syndrome in unselected Caucasian women from Spain1. The Journal of Clinical Endocrinology & Metabolism. 2000;**85**:2434-2438

[2] Nandi A, Chen Z, Patel R, Poretsky L. Polycystic ovary syndrome. Endocrinology and Metabolism Clinics of North America. 2014;**43**:123-147

[3] Tamaddon M, Azimzadeh M, Tavangar SM. microRNAs and long non-coding RNAs as biomarkers for polycystic ovary syndrome. Journal of Cellular and Molecular Medicine. 2022;**26**:654-670

[4] Taft RJ, Pheasant M, Mattick JS. The relationship between non-protein-coding DNA and eukaryotic complexity. BioEssays. 2007;**29**:288-299

[5] Wang XY, Qin YY. Long non-coding RNAs in biology and female reproductive disorders. Frontiers in Biosciences (Landmark Ed). 2019;**24**:750-764

[6] Abolghasemi M, Mahjoub S. Long noncoding RNAs as a piece of polycystic ovary syndrome puzzle. Molecular Biology Reports. 2021;**48**:3845-3851

[7] Mu L, Sun X, Tu M, Zhang D. Non-coding RNAs in polycystic ovary syndrome: A systematic review and meta-analysis. Reproductive Biology and Endocrinology. 2021;**19**:10

[8] Zhang R, Wesevich V, Chen Z, Zhang D, Kallen AN. Emerging roles for noncoding RNAs in female sex steroids and reproductive disease. Molecular and Cellular Endocrinology. 2020;**518**:110875

[9] Zhou Z, Zhang Y, Tan C, Zhang J, Yi G, Wang B, et al. The long non-coding RNA BBOX1 antisense RNA 1 is upregulated in polycystic ovary syndrome (PCOS) and suppresses the role of microRNA-19b in the proliferation of ovarian granulose cells. BMC Women's Health. 2023;**23**:508

[10] Tu M, Wu Y, Mu L, Zhang D. Long non-coding RNAs: Novel players in the pathogenesis of polycystic ovary syndrome. Annals of Translational Medicine. 2021;**9**:173

[11] Kamalidehghan B, Habibi M, Afjeh SS, Shoai M, Alidoost S, Almasi Ghale R, et al. The importance of small non-coding RNAs in human reproduction: A review article. The Application of Clinical Genetics. 2020;**13**:1-11

[12] Robles V, Valcarce DG, Riesco MF. Non-coding RNA regulation in reproduction: Their potential use as biomarkers. Noncoding RNA Research. 2019;**4**:54-62

[13] De Leo V, Musacchio MC, Cappelli V, Massaro MG, Morgante G, Petraglia F. Genetic, hormonal and metabolic aspects of PCOS: An update. Reproductive Biology and Endocrinology. 2016;**14**:38

[14] Abdalla M, Deshmukh H, Atkin SL, Sathyapalan T. miRNAs as a novel clinical biomarker and therapeutic targets in polycystic ovary syndrome (PCOS): A review. Life Sciences. 2020;**259**:118174

[15] Sørensen AE, Wissing ML, Englund ALM, Dalgaard LT. MicroRNA species in follicular fluid associating with polycystic ovary syndrome and related intermediary phenotypes. The Journal of Clinical Endocrinology & Metabolism. 2016;**101**:1579-1589

[16] Apparao K, Lovely LP, Gui Y, Lininger RA, Lessey BA. Elevated endometrial androgen receptor expression in women with polycystic ovarian syndrome. Biology of Reproduction. 2002;**66**:297-304

[17] Chen Z, Liu L, Xi X, Burn M, Karakaya C, Kallen AN. Aberrant H19 expression disrupts ovarian Cyp17 and testosterone production and is associated with polycystic ovary syndrome in women. Reproductive Sciences. 2022;**29**:1357-1367

[18] Wickham EP 3rd, Tao T, Nestler JE, McGee EA. Activation of the LH receptor up regulates the type 2 adiponectin receptor in human granulosa cells. Journal of Assisted Reproduction and Genetics. 2013;**30**:963-968

[19] Song J, Luo S, Li SW. miRNA-592 is downregulated and may target LHCGR in polycystic ovary syndrome patients. Reproductive Biology. 2015;**15**:229-237

[20] Zhang X, Xiao H, Zhang X, Gong X, Li T, Han Y, et al. Decreased microRNA-125b-5p disrupts follicle steroidogenesis through targeting PAK3/ERK1/2 signalling in mouse preantral follicles. Metabolism. 2020;**107**:154241

[21] Gebremedhn S, Ali A, Hossain M, Hoelker M, Salilew-Wondim D, Anthony RV, et al. MicroRNA-mediated gene regulatory mechanisms in mammalian female reproductive health. International Journal of Molecular Sciences. 2021;**22**:938

[22] Xiong W, Lin Y, Xu L, Tamadon A, Zou S, Tian F, et al. Circulatory microRNA 23a and microRNA 23b and polycystic ovary syndrome (PCOS): The effects of body mass index and sex hormones in an Eastern Han Chinese population. Journal of Ovarian Research. 2017;**10**

[23] Xu S, Linher-Melville K, Yang BB, Wu D, Li J. Micro-RNA378 (miR-378) regulates ovarian estradiol production by targeting aromatase. Endocrinology. 2011;**152**:3941-3951

[24] Zhang Q, Sun H, Jiang Y, Ding L, Wu S, Fang T, et al. MicroRNA-181a suppresses mouse granulosa cell proliferation by targeting activin receptor IIA. PLoS One. 2013;**8**:e59667

[25] Butler AE, Ramachandran V, Hayat S, Dargham SR, Cunningham TK, Benurwar M, et al. Expression of microRNA in follicular fluid in women with and without PCOS. Scientific Reports. 2019;**9**:16306

[26] Liu Y, Zhang S, Chen L, Huang X, Wang M, Ponikwicka-Tyszko D, et al. The molecular mechanism of miR-96-5p in the pathogenesis and treatment of polycystic ovary syndrome. Translational Research. 2023;**256**:1-13

[27] Xue Y, Lv J, Xu P, Gu L, Cao J, Xu L, et al. Identification of microRNAs and genes associated with hyperandrogenism in the follicular fluid of women with polycystic ovary syndrome. Journal of Cellular Biochemistry. 2018;**119**:3913-3921

[28] Yin M, Wang X, Yao G, Lü M, Liang M, Sun Y, et al. Transactivation of micrornA-320 by microRNA-383 regulates granulosa cell functions by targeting E2F1 and SF-1 proteins. The Journal of Biological Chemistry. 2014;**289**:18239-18257

[29] Sang Q, Yao Z, Wang H, Feng R, Wang H, Zhao X, et al. Identification of microRNAs in human follicular fluid: Characterization of microRNAs that govern steroidogenesis in vitro and are associated with polycystic ovary syndrome *in vivo*. The Journal of Clinical Endocrinology & Metabolism. 2013;**98**:3068-3079

[30] Che Q, Liu M, Zhang D, Lu Y, Xu J, Lu X, et al. Long noncoding RNA HUPCOS promotes follicular fluid androgen excess in PCOS patients via aromatase inhibition. The Journal of Clinical Endocrinology and Metabolism. 2020;**105**:dgaa060

[31] Wu G, Yang Z, Chen Y, Li X, Yang J, Yin T. Downregulation of Lnc-OC1 attenuates the pathogenesis of polycystic ovary syndrome. Molecular and Cellular Endocrinology. 2020;**506**:110760

[32] Zhu H-L, Chen Y-Q, Zhang Z-F. Downregulation of lncRNA ZFAS1 and upregulation of microRNA-129 repress endocrine disturbance, increase proliferation and inhibit apoptosis of ovarian granulosa cells in polycystic ovarian syndrome by downregulating HMGB1. Genomics. 2020;**112**:3597-3608

[33] Nasser JS, Altahoo N, Almosawi S, Alhermi A, Butler AE. The role of MicroRNA, long non-coding RNA and circular RNA in the pathogenesis of polycystic ovary syndrome: A literature review. International Journal of Molecular Sciences. 2024;**25**:903

[34] Zhao J, Huang J, Geng X, Chu W, Li S, Chen Z-J, et al. Polycystic ovary syndrome: Novel and hub lncRNAs in the insulin resistance-associated lncRNA–mRNA network. Frontiers in Genetics. 2019;**10**:772

[35] Diamanti-Kandarakis E, Christakou CD. Insulin resistance in PCOS. In: Diagnosis and Management of Polycystic Ovary Syndrome. Endocrine (Springer Science & Business Media). Aug 2006;**30**(1):13-17. DOI: 10.1385/ENDO:30:1:13. PMID: 17185787

[36] Sathyapalan T, David R, Gooderham NJ, Atkin SL. Increased expression of circulating miRNA-93 in women with polycystic ovary syndrome may represent a novel, non-invasive biomarker for diagnosis. Scientific Reports. 2015;**5**:16890

[37] Long W, Zhao C, Ji C, Ding H, Cui Y, Guo X, et al. Characterization of serum microRNAs profile of PCOS and identification of novel non-invasive biomarkers. Cellular Physiology and Biochemistry. 2014;**33**:1304-1315

[38] Balasubramanyam M, Aravind S, Gokulakrishnan K, Prabu P, Sathishkumar C, Ranjani H, et al. Impaired miR-146a expression links subclinical inflammation and insulin resistance in type 2 diabetes. Molecular and Cellular Biochemistry. 2011;**351**:197-205

[39] Chen Y-H, Heneidi S, Lee J-M, Layman LC, Stepp DW, Gamboa GM, et al. miRNA-93 inhibits GLUT4 and is overexpressed in adipose tissue of polycystic ovary syndrome patients and women with insulin resistance. Diabetes. 2013;**62**:2278-2286

[40] Angioni S, Sanna S, Magnini R, Melis GB, Fulghesu AM. The quantitative insulin sensitivity check index is not able to detect early metabolic alterations in young patients with polycystic ovarian syndrome. Gynecological Endocrinology. 2011;**27**:468-474

[41] Capuani B, Pacifici F, Della-Morte D, Lauro D. Glucagon like peptide 1 and MicroRNA in metabolic diseases: Focusing on GLP1 action on miRNAs. Frontiers in Endocrinology (Lausanne). 2018;**9**:719

[42] Radbakhsh S, Sathyapalan T, Banach M, Sahebkar A. Incretins and microRNAs: Interactions and physiological relevance. Pharmacological Research. 2020;**153**:104662

[43] Cao J, Huo P, Cui K, Wei H, Cao J, Wang J, et al. Follicular fluid-derived exosomal miR-143-3p/miR-155-5p regulate follicular dysplasia by modulating glycolysis in granulosa cells in polycystic ovary syndrome. Cell Communication and Signaling. 2022;**20**:61

[44] Chakraborty C, Doss CGP, Bandyopadhyay S, Agoramoorthy G. Influence of miRNA in insulin signaling pathway and insulin resistance: Micro-molecules with a major role in type-2 diabetes. Wiley Interdisciplinary Reviews: RNA. 2014;**5**:697-712

[45] Cai G, Ma X, Chen B, Huang Y, Liu S, Yang H, et al. MicroRNA-145 negatively regulates cell proliferation through targeting IRS1 in isolated ovarian granulosa cells from patients with polycystic ovary syndrome. Reproductive Sciences. 2017;**24**:902-910

[46] Mao Z, Fan L, Yu Q, Luo S, Wu X, Tang J, et al. Abnormality of klotho signaling is involved in polycystic ovary syndrome. Reproductive Sciences. 2017;**25**:372-383

[47] Gao L, Wu D, Wu Y, Yang Z, Sheng J, Lin X, et al. MiR-3940-5p promotes granulosa cell proliferation through targeting KCNA5 in polycystic ovarian syndrome. Biochemical and Biophysical Research Communications. 2020;**524**:791-797

[48] Pei C-Z, Jin L, Baek K-H. Pathogenetic analysis of polycystic ovary syndrome from the perspective of omics. Biomedicine & Pharmacotherapy. 2021;**142**:112031

[49] Shi L, Liu S, Zhao W, Shi J. miR-483-5p and miR-486-5p are down-regulated in cumulus cells of metaphase II oocytes from women with polycystic ovary syndrome. Reproductive Biomedicine Online. 2015;**31**:565-572

[50] Xu B, Zhang Y-W, Tong X-H, Liu Y-S. Characterization of microRNA profile in human cumulus granulosa cells: Identification of microRNAs that regulate notch signaling and are associated with PCOS. Molecular and Cellular Endocrinology. 2015;**404**:26-36

[51] Zhang C-L, Wang H, Yan C-Y, Gao X-F, Ling X-J. Deregulation of RUNX2 by miR-320a deficiency impairs steroidogenesis in cumulus granulosa cells from polycystic ovary syndrome (PCOS) patients. Biochemical and Biophysical Research Communications. 2017;**482**:1469-1476

[52] Jiang L, Huang J, Chen Y, Yang Y, Li R, Li Y, et al. Identification of several circulating microRNAs from a genome-wide circulating microRNA expression profile as potential biomarkers for impaired glucose metabolism in polycystic ovarian syndrome. Endocrine. 2016;**53**:280-290

[53] He T, Liu Y, Jia Y, Wang H, Yang X, Lu G, et al. MicroRNA-141 and MicroRNA-200c are overexpressed in granulosa cells of polycystic ovary syndrome patients. Frontiers in Medicine. 2018;**5**:299

[54] Huang X, Hao C, Bao H, Wang M, Dai H. Aberrant expression of long noncoding RNAs in cumulus cells isolated from PCOS patients. Journal of Assisted Reproduction and Genetics. 2016;**33**:111-121

[55] Liu S, Zhang X, Shi C, Lin J, Chen G, Wu B, et al. Altered microRNAs expression profiling in cumulus cells from patients with polycystic ovary syndrome. Journal of Translational Medicine. 2015;**13**:238

[56] Liu Z, Hao C, Song D, Zhang N, Bao H, Qu Q. Androgen receptor coregulator CTBP1-AS is associated

with polycystic ovary syndrome in Chinese women: A preliminary study. Reproductive Sciences. 2015;**22**:829-837

[57] Chen S, Ren C, Zheng H, Sun X, Dai J. The effect of long non-coding RNA (lncRNA) HCP5 on regulating epithelial-mesenchymal transition (EMT)-related markers in gastric carcinoma is partially reversed by miR-27b-3p. Medical Science Monitor. 2020;**26**:e921383

[58] Gao H, Jiang J, Shi Y, Chen J, Zhao L, Wang C. The LINC00477/miR-128 axis promotes the progression of polycystic ovary syndrome by regulating ovarian granulosa cell proliferation and apoptosis. Reproductive Biology and Endocrinology. 2021;**19**:29

[59] Li Y, Zhang J, Liu Y-D, Zhou X-Y, Chen X, Zhe J, et al. Long non-coding RNA TUG1 and its molecular mechanisms in polycystic ovary syndrome. RNA Biology. 2020;**17**:1798-1810

[60] Liu Y-D, Li Y, Feng S-X, Ye D-S, Chen X, Zhou X-Y, et al. Long noncoding RNAs: Potential regulators involved in the pathogenesis of polycystic ovary syndrome. Endocrinology. 2017;**158**:3890-3899

[61] Zeng Z, Lin X, Xia T, Liu W, Tian X, Li M. Identification of crucial lncRNAs, miRNAs, mRNAs, and potential therapeutic compounds for polycystic ovary syndrome by bioinformatics analysis. BioMed Research International. 2020;**2020**:1817094

[62] Huang J, Zhao J, Geng X, Chu W, Li S, Chen Z-J, et al. Long non-coding RNA lnc-CCNL1-3:1 promotes granulosa cell apoptosis and suppresses glucose uptake in women with polycystic ovary syndrome. Molecular Therapy-Nucleic Acids. 2021;**23**:614-628

Section 3

Polycystic Ovary Syndrome Treatment

Chapter 5

Effects of Acupuncture Treatment on Polycystic Ovary Syndrome (PCOS)

Gunasekaran Ramanathan

Abstract

Polycystic ovarian syndrome (PCOS) is an imbalance of endocrine hormones with a group of symptoms that occur in the reproductive age of females. It is diagnosed by androgen excess and ovarian dysfunction. Many pharmacological-based drugs and treatments are available, however, the effectiveness of existing therapies is less. Yet no cure for PCOS, but symptoms can be managed with medications and lifestyle modifications. Hence, an alternative treatment method is needed for a complete cure. Currently, much clinical evidence has revealed that Acupuncture (AP) and Electro-acupuncture treatment (EAT) are effective treatments for regulating reproductive hormone levels, normalizing testosterone, reducing ovarian cysts, enhancing ovulation, and weakening insulin resistance in normal and obese women with PCOS. Further, β-endorphin has a more crucial role in PCO, AP, or EAT, which may alter the formation of β-endorphin. The mechanism of AP and EAT for PCOS has not been widely reviewed so far. A good understanding of the AP and EAT would be helpful in women with PCOS. This chapter aimed to overview the probable mechanisms and experimental evidence-based data of acupuncture treatment on PCOS in animal models and human patients. We hope that the chapter study will contribute to a better understanding of the PCOS and AP treatment.

Keywords: acupuncture, electro-acupuncture treatment, PCOS, anovulation, ovarian cysts anovulation, HR variability

1. Introduction

Polycystic ovary syndrome (PCOS) is an endocrine disorder. In the modern lifestyle, the disorder affects many reproductive-age women worldwide. In 2010 data worldwide, 116 million (3.42%) women were affected by PCOS [1]. PCO is majorly associated with the dysfunction of ovaries. Based on studies, many factors are involved. The clinical signs of PCO are hyperandrogenism, ovulatory dysfunction, metabolic dysfunction, and obesity [2, 3] further, it is associated with cardiovascular disease CVD, cancer, diabetes, and endometrial dysfunction [4, 5], but the exact cause, etiology, and pathophysiology are not clearly understood. Yet there is no perfect treatment for all diagnosed with PCOS [6, 7]. Depending on the patient, the PCO management method and selection of the best therapy option and their priorities vary [8, 9].

The current management, therapy, and pharmacological medications are less effective in PCOS, yet some complicated women with PCOS are left untreated [10]. Currently, the pharmacological therapy for women with PCOS is using an oral estrogen receptor modulator, but it's 40–50% ineffective in many cases. It's linked with side effects such as breast tenderness, headaches, mood swings, arthralgias, myalgias, and fatigue [11, 12]. Further studies showed pituitary Gonadotropin (GnH) hormone is effective in inducing ovulation; however, it causes overstimulation syndrome and the development of multiple follicles [13].

Recent research showed that complementary and alternative medicine (CAM) as alternative therapy might benefit the management of PCOS [14]. The CAM therapeutic input has classes of physical, nutritional, and psychological, or all in combination [15]. Hence, clear-cut PCOS pathogenesis and perfect management are urgently needed. In this book chapter, we update the pathogenesis and current management, particularly the beneficial effects of electro-acupuncture on PCOS.

2. What is acupuncture treatment?

Acupuncture has origins in traditional Chinese medicine (TCM) [16], More than 3000 years, ago acupuncture treatment was used; it's a basic part of CAM [14] acupuncture is a specific type of sensory stimulation in the skin and muscles using thin needles. It may be useful to treat some chronic pain, and some abnormal physical conditions, and as a complementary treatment for many disorders [17].

3. How is acupuncture working?

TCM describes that a person's health results from a tuneful balance of the complementary extremes of Chinese Yin and Yang of the life force known as Qi marked "chi." It believes that disease is the result of an imbalance of these forces. In the human body, the Qi flows through specific pathways, or meridians. These energy flows and pathways are accessible through specific acupuncture points. In the human body 361, acupuncture points have been identified. Inserting selected thin needles into these suitable acupoints with suitable combinations will bring the flow of energy back into balance [18].

Stimulation of many acupuncture points affects multiple sensory neuron activity. These points are called the receptive fields. The physical insertion of a thin needle may affect pain processing in the muscles and central nervous system (CNS), further increasing blood flow to certain organs and parts of the body [19]. However, the exact mechanism of action of acupuncture is not clear.

4. What's electro-acupuncture treatment (EAT)?

In China1950s EAT was developed for its precise use in surgical operations. In the early days, acupuncture was used for analgesia; while using it, the anesthetists had to rotate the needles manually throughout the surgery, which was difficult, so they developed an electro-acupuncture (EA) apparatus. EAT, in which acupuncture is united with electrical stimulation. Initially, EA analgesia was used largely in China, and interest showed in the West. It's useful to reduce the use of analgesic drugs during surgery. However, EA in practice is personal and depends on their experience. Some practitioners said EA is against the spirit of 'natural' acupuncture therapy, but others said EAT is good for patients with chronic nociceptive pain and good for drug addiction.

The analgesic effects of EAT are more effective than those of the manual acupuncture method. An fMRI study of normal adults found that stimulation with EA at a frequency of 3 Hz on acupuncture point LI-4 Hegu produced fMRI signal increases in the precentral gyrus, postcentral gyrus/inferior parietal lobule, and putamen/insula [20], whereas normal acupuncture through specific needle manipulation manually of the same acupuncture point produced decreases in fMRI signals in the putamen/insula, posterior cingulate, and superior temporal gyrus [21]. EA also increases the tissue content of endorphins [22].

Electro-acupuncture (EA) can be used for seizures, dizziness, aphasia, headache, chorea, stroke, drug addiction, PCO, and many more. Currently, two modes of EA are used commonly: high-intensity high-frequency (50 to 200 Hz) and low-intensity low-frequency (1 to 4 Hz). In this EA therapy, instead of hand stimulation through a needle, electro-stimulation is used to treat the diseases. In EAT-specific needles are placed in the scalp (anastomotic linkage of lymphatic drainage) and connected with an electro-acupuncture machine to stimulate the acupuncture points. The pulse duration, intensity, and frequency of the electric current must be altered depending on the patient. EAT stabilizes the treatment through its fast rotation; we can stimulate more than two points simultaneously and control the current level depending on the patient. Usually, EAT duration is 10 to 20 minutes per time for 7–10 days depending on the disease.

EAT should be used with caution. Use the needle in the right position, not bend or break. When the intensity of the current used for acupuncture points close to the brain area, medulla, lateral line of the occipital area, or other areas, at all times the right amount of current must be used. Do not increase the current suddenly to a large amount because it may cause an increase in heart rate (HR) and breathing stops. It's contraindicated for cancer, heart diseases, and brain diseases.

5. Electroacupuncture treatment for PCOS

Conventional therapy (first-line) is not yet satisfactory, but the nonpharmacological therapy of normal acupuncture and EA has become popular. Based on multiple clinical trials, both manual acupuncture and EAT have a good effect on treating women with PCO [23–27]. Earlier studies and clinical trials suggested that proper acupuncture treatment improves menstruation and ovulation [28, 29]. It has also been reported that EAT decreases testosterone levels and improves insulin sensitivity in animals and humans with PCOS [23]. Further, it regulates the levels of the anti-Müllerian hormone (AMH) and hypothalamic–pituitary-ovarian (HPO) axis. A recent animal models PCO study explain that acupuncture could improve insulin resistance inhibit the PI3K/AKT/mTOR pathway, or activate the protein kinase (AMPK) pathway [30]. Further, it reduces anxiety and improves

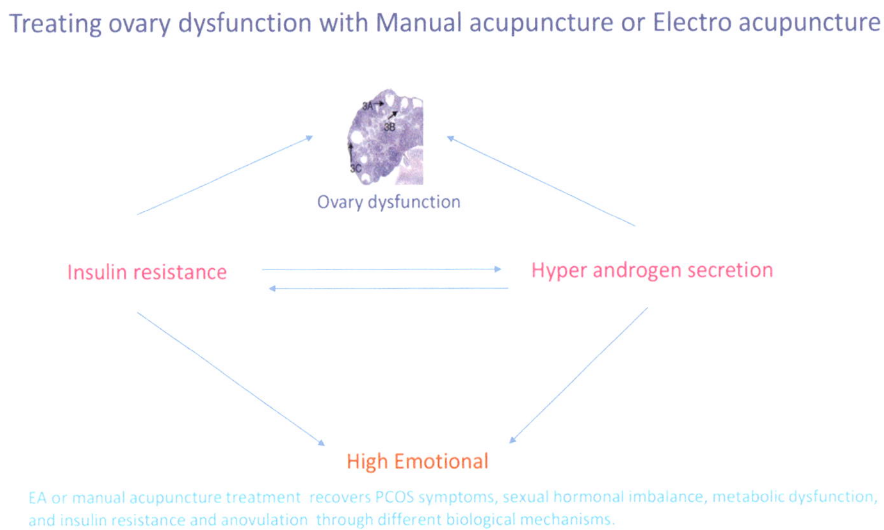

Figure 1.
Manual or EAT improves PCOS-related symptoms such as pregnancy rate, ovulation rate, sexual hormonal imbalance, metabolic dysfunction, and insulin resistance through different biological mechanisms.

health-related quality of life [31]. Acupuncture treatment for patients with PCOS decreases the abnormally increased luteinizing hormone (LH) [29, 32] and increased testosterone [33] without side effects; it's less expensive treatment [34]. Collectively, the manual or EAT for PCOs improves the pregnancy rate. Ovulation rate, sexual hormonal imbalance, metabolic dysfunction, and insulin resistance (**Figure 1**).

6. Methods of electroacupuncture treatment

Stimulation through EA is more effective and can be easily quantifiable compared to manual acupuncture, further reducing the bias. Earlier studies showed Zigong (EX-CA 1), Sanyinjiao (SP 6), Zhongji (CV 3), and Guanyuan (BL 26) acupuncture points were chosen for the formula. In addition to that, three arbitrary acupuncture points have been selected based on phases of the menstrual cycle: 1) after menstruation, using acupuncture points for the needle: Taixi (KI 3) and Taichong (LR 3). 2) In the ovulatory period, using acupuncture points: Xuehai (SP 10) and Mingmen (CV 4). 3) Using acupuncture points before the beginning of the next menstruation: Geshu (BL 17) and Xuehai (SP 10).

The broadly used acupuncture point was SP6 (Sanyinjiao) for reproductive problems, nourishing organs, and activating blood; the second ST29 (Guilai) acupoint was used for reducing pain and regulating circulation and menstruation. An EAT, or manual acupuncture needle stimulation, induces and enhances muscle conduction and various chemical signals to stimulate the central release of various factors through sympathetic nerve conduction, which is believed to regulate the woman's reproductive axis (**Figure 2**).

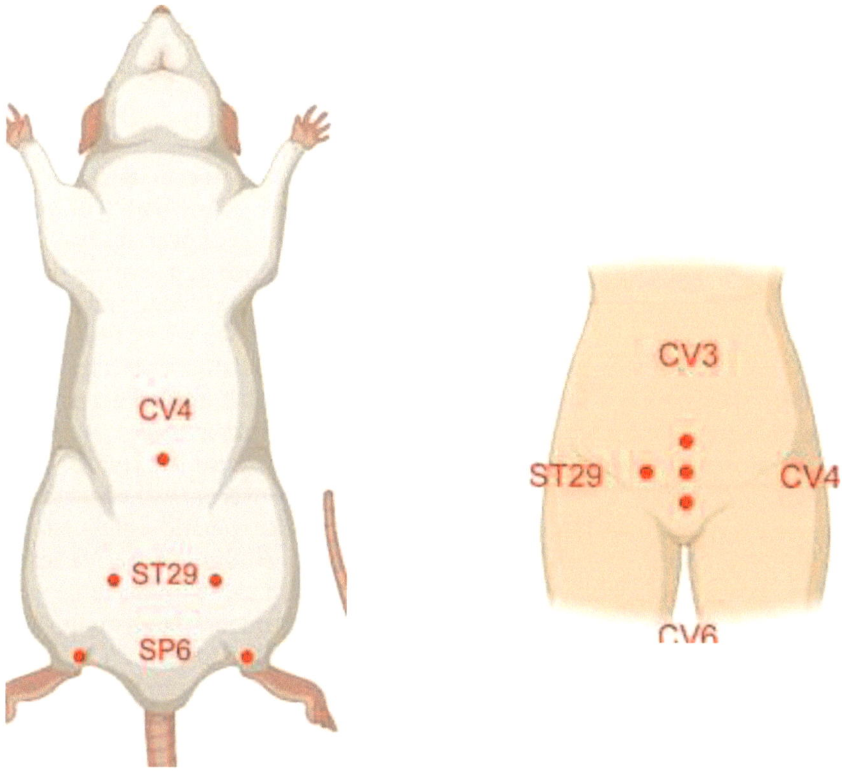

Figure 2.
The most of the acupuncture needle points are on the abdominal area for human and animal for PCO, the acupuncture point SP6 (Sanyinjiao)for reproductive problem, nourishing organs, and activating blood. The acupuncture point ST29 (Guilai) was used for reducing pain and regulate menstruation.

7. Needle using

An earlier study [35] showed that each acupuncture point needled used a filiform needle (length 25–50 mm and diameter 0.25–026 mm) to attain a *Deqi* sensation3 (at the needling acupuncture point, feel a sensation like numbness and swelling, and it radiates along the reliable meridian). Needled used in each acupuncture point will be a filiform needle (length 25–50 mm and diameter 0.25 mm) to achieve a *Deqi* sensation. Then, an auxiliary needle (length: 13 mm and diameter: 0.18 mm) will be inserted to a depth of 2 mm and 2 mm lateral to the first needle without achieving *Deqi*.4. With the help of an EA instrument, fixed or required electrical current will be given at the acupuncture point, with one electrode to the auxiliary and the other electrode to the filiform needle [35].

Duration of treatment: Electrical stimulation for a minimum of 30 min for each session. From the 50th day of menstruation three times per week or withdrawal bleeding until before the next menstruation for three menstrual cycles.

Expected outcome: Primary outcome: the ovulation rate. Secondary outcomes: ovulation time point, endometrial thickness, dominant follicle rate, and follicular size Hormone level: FSH, LH, GnRH, Estradiol (E2) level, and pregnancy rate.

8. EAT rectifies the anovulation in PCO

8.1 Experimental evidence

Experimental evidence PCOS is a complex metabolic and endocrine disorder [36]. In the reproductive age of females, many cases of anovulation occur, which leads to infertility. EA treatment is a safe and effective treatment for anovulation in women 5A suitable EA treatment may effectively reduce the number of ovarian cysts, reduce ovarian volume, and enhance blood flow to the ovaries. Further, it reverses the insulin levels and insulin sensitivity back to normal, which reduces the blood glucose level. Further, it controls the sympathetic activity to normal [37]. Only very few animal model studies are available on the effect of EAT on the sympathetic activity in PCOS. Hence, in our laboratory, we aimed to assess the effect of EAT on anovulation and increased sympathetic nerve activity in EV-induced PCO rate models.

EAT: Repeated low-frequency EAT was carried out for 20 minutes for the PCO group for two days up to 8–10 weeks. Just before EAT rats were anesthetized, the needles were inserted into the erector spinae muscle in the somatic segment and bilaterally in the biceps femoris related to the nerve innervations of the ovaries, inserted to a depth of 0.3–0.51 cm. 6 These are connected to the EA machine using the frequencies of 80 Hz (burst frequency) and 2 Hz (frequency low), and until local muscle contraction, the intensity was adjusted to be from 0.8 to 1.31 mA. After the experimental period, animals were anesthetized and the blood samples were collected to measure plasma epinephrine (EPI) and norepinephrine (NE) levels in high-performance liquid chromatography (HPLC).

8.2 Histological study of the ovaries

For the histological study of ovaries, the control and experimental groups were euthanized, ovaries were removed, and the near connective fat tissue was removed. The tissue sections were stained with hematoxylin–eosin (NICE chemicals), and then the slides were used to study the follicles. The slides were viewed under a light microscope, and a well-trained pathologist determined the morphological variation of the normal and abnormal follicles in the follicular population. In this case, a normal ovary has become a polycystic ovary (PCO). We can see on the outer border of the ovary many small fluid-filled sacs present. These sacs are called cysts, which contain immature eggs. The cystic follicle's failure to release eggs leads to anovulation.

Most of the follicles are cystic in appearance, and stromal hyperplasia was seen. Follicles become atretic; otherwise, the ovary and follicles were considered healthy.

We got the following result: After the experimental period of 30, and 60 days, the normal, EV-induced PCO and EA treatment rates were killed. After 30 days, PCO rates showed a progressive decline in the number of primary and secondary follicles, but after 60 days, there were many morphological variations seen in the PCO rat's follicles compared to normal healthy follicles, and follicular cysts appeared, big-size atretic follicles, and stromal hyperplasia were also seen. It confirms that the ovary attains PCOS (**Figure 3B**) similar result was also observed in an earlier study [38]. Repeated EAT after 60 days showed the abnormal follicle morphology back to normal and the number of ovarian cysts considerably reducing (**Figure 3C**). Furthermore, no considerable morphological differences were seen between the healthy rats ovary (Control group **Figure 3A**) and the EAT group rats' ovary (**Figure 3**).

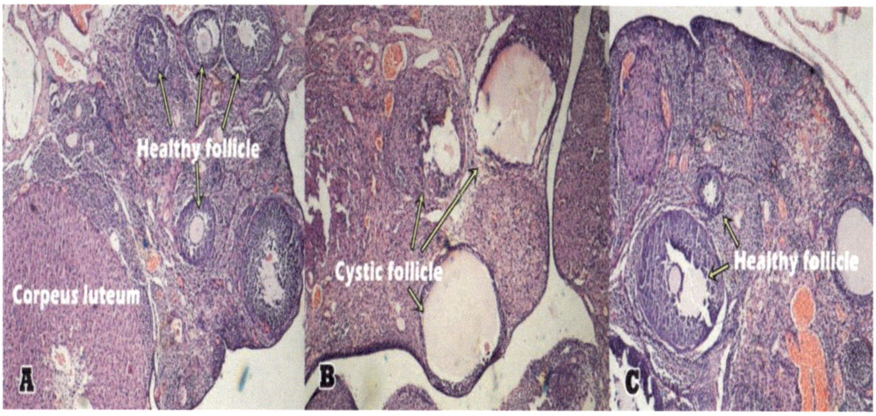

Figure 3.
Hematoxylin and eosin-stained ovary section. A. The normal control rats ovaries with healthy follicles and corpus luteum, B. EV-induced rat's ovaries showed cystic appearance, and C. After electroacupuncture treatment in PCOS rats showed reappearance of healthy follicles.

8.3 Epinephrine and norepinephrine levels in rat plasma

In our study, the EV-treated PCO rats showed a significant increase in the epinephrine (EPI) and norepinephrine (NE), but after 60 days of EAT, the PCO group rates showed a significant decrease in both EPI and NE levels ($P < 0.001$). When it's compared to the control group with the EAT group, the EPI and NE levels are back to normal (**Table 1**).

Parameters	Normal control ng/ml Mean + SD	PCO before EAT ng/ml Mean + SD	PCO after EAT ng/ml Mean + SD	P value
Epinephrine	0.257 + 0.04903	0.41190 + .03924	0.26001 + .05191	P < 0.001
Norepinephrine	0.2386+ 0.05797	0.3994 + 0.05425	0.25821 + 0.04945	P < 0.001

Table 1.
Epinephrine and norepinephrine level in rat plasma (Normal and PCO, EAT).

9. The potential mechanisms of EAT and anovulation

Chronic anovulation is a main cause of infertility; in both animals and humans, anovulation is the supreme characteristic of PCOS [39]. EAT improves the development and maturation of follicles and oocytes and prevents anovulation [26, 40]. It's by increasing the expression of P450arom, inhibiting the overexpression of, and upregulating the IRS-1/PI3K/GLUT4 pathway. Further, EA improved *in vitro* fertilization [41]. Various animal model studies also reported that EA improves ovulation dysfunction by reducing granulosa atrophy, improving follicular arrest, inhibiting the PI3K/AKT/mTOR pathway, and downregulating LncMEG3 expression [42, 43]. EAT also improves the preovulatory follicle number and development of corporalutea. It's by increasing the hilum blood vessels and blood supply [44].

In women, a range of reproductive hormonal disturbances cause PCO. EAT rectifies the hormonal imbalance of decreased GnRH, estradiol, and increased LH in women with PCO [45]. Acupuncture reduces the abnormal serum sex steroid levels of the adrenal cortex and ovaries. In the PCO animal model study, EAT improved the number of corpora lutea, disturbed estrous cycles, and upregulated the arcuate nucleus kisspeptin protein [46].

10. EAT rectifies the autonomic alteration in women with PCOS

10.1 Experimental evidence

Heart rate (HR) fluctuation is a sign of autonomic imbalance. Based on earlier studies, it's an initial risk for heart problems, and it may lead to CVD. Further, studies showed that a group of PCOS women has a risk of CVD [4]. Therefore, in our laboratory, we aimed to investigate the autonomic alteration of the HR in women with PCOS and the effect of EAT on it. For this study, we used the estradiol valerate (EV)-induced PCO rat model [47]. In this study, the vaginal smear was taken periodically from the control and experimental group rats. The EV-induced PCO model rat group shows a prolonged diestrus stage compared to the control group; we determine its PCO group rat [47].

Heart rate variability (HRV) analysis: Our laboratory's heart rate variability (HRV) was assessed in the normal control group and experimental PCO group rats before and after EAT. It's done from the frequency domain and the time domain analysis. In the time domain analysis, the following data were obtained: mean RR interval, SDNN (standard deviation of RR interval), and rMSSD. For frequency domain analysis, there were two major spectral components: high frequency (HF 0.8–2.5 Hz) and low frequency (LF 0.2–0.8 Hz).

EAT: For this study, we carried out low-frequency EAT in the conformed PCOS rats; each treatment was given once in two days for 15–20 minutes, given up to 4–5 weeks. The EA needles were inserted in the erector spinae muscle in the somatic segment and bilaterally in the biceps femoris related to the nerve innervations of the ovaries, with a needle depth of 0.3–0.5 cm. Then it connected to an EA electrical stimulator with a burst frequency of 80 Hz and a low frequency of 2 Hz.

The result obtained: The EV-induced PCO rate showed a significant reduction ($p < 0.05$). in the time domain R-R interval, SDNN, and rMSSD compared to the control group, but after 4–5 weeks of EAT, the PCO group rats showed a significant increase in the R-R interval, SDNN, and rMSSD ($p < 0.05$). It indicates that the repeated low frequency EAT has beneficial effects on PCOS rats; the RR interval and HR significantly returned to normal (**Table 2**).

Parameters	Control	PCO	EAT
Mean RR	176 ± 3.9	150 ± 3.9*	170.7 ± 3.3**
SDNN	13.6 ± 1.5	10.76 ± 1.5*	11.6 ± 0.8
rMSSD	5.8 ± 0.9	3.46 ± 0.69*	5.5 ± 0.9**

In comparison with the control group the PCO group showed a significant decrease ($p < 0.05$). And comparison with the PCOS group with PCO + EAT showed a significant increase ($p < 0.05$)**.*

Table 2.
The control group, PCO, and PCO + EAT groups were compared in time domain indices the values are in mean ± SD.

The frequency domain analysis of the PCOS rats showed a significant increase in the low-frequency power LF and LF/ HF ratio. But total power TP ($p < 0.05$) and high-frequency power HF, when compared to control, significantly decreased. However, after 4–5 weeks of EAT, the LF and LF/HF ratios significantly decreased and the HF and TP increased when compared to untreated PCOS (**Table 3**).

10.2 Mechanisms EAT on HR variability in PCO

In our study, short-term HRV analysis of the EV-induced PCO rat showed a significant decrease in the total power (TP), which is an index of overall HRV. A further significant increase in LF nu showed increased sympathetic activity, and a significantly decreased HF nu indicates decreased parasympathetic activity. Furthermore, the LF/HF ratio also increased, which indicates an imbalance between sympathetic nerve and parasympathetic nerve activity. Earlier studies also showed an increase in LF and LF/HF ratio, which is due to increased sympathetic activity [48]. In another study, EV-induced PCO model rats significantly increased the synthesis of intra-ovarian nerve growth factor (NGF), which is a strong marker for sympathetic activity [49]. Increased activity of sympathetic nerves is also linked with obesity and CVD [50, 51]. In a comparative study, PCOS was treated with exercise with low-frequency EAT, which has shown significantly decreased high muscle sympathetic activity [52]. In the EV-induced PCOS, model rats showed the EAT decreased the high ovarian NGF and high mRNA expression of NGF [37, 53, 54] and adrenergic receptors [55].

10.3 The mechanisms of acupuncture treatment on hyperandrogenism

Hyperandrogenism is a condition in which overproduction of the male sex hormone (testosterone), even though these hormones are present in women at lower levels. But in some women, excess levels of male sex hormones androsterone, androstenedione, and testosterone causes Cushing syndrome, PCO, and malfunction of the adrenal gland. Erlaier's studies showed that hyperandrogenism is the most important mechanism and clinical feature of PCOS [56]. EAT normalizes the blood testosterone level in women with PCOs [28]. Further, in the rate model PCO, the low-frequency EAT also reduces the serum androgen level through the hypothalamic *Oprk1* and *Oprm1* central opioid receptors [57]. In another study in PCO women, EAT regulates the AMH and P450arom through this mechanism, it reduces the increased androgen level [58]. A similar result was also observed in the rat model PCO study by Sun et al. [59]. Another PCO animal model study also reveals that acupuncture treatment reduces abnormally increased androgen secretion and reduces the number of androgen receptors [60].

Parameters	Control group	PCO group	PCO+ EAT group
HF	15.87 ± 4.04	8.62 ± 0.7*	3.7 ± 2.07**
LF	15.07 ± 1.8	20.32 ± 2.5*	16.5 ± 1.7**
LF/HF	0.98 ± 0.18	1.72 ± 0.17*	1.2 ± 0.18**
TP	71.6 ± 10.3	41.75 ± 6.9*	65.8 ± 11.3**

Table 3.
*The frequency domain analysis comparison between groups * and ** indicates significant.*

10.4 Obesity and PCO

Obesity has increased the amount of body fat and is a complex disease. It's the root of many diseases and health problems like diabetes, high cholesterol, heart disease, high blood pressure, and liver disease. Its comorbidity is associated with cardiometabolic dysfunction like hypertension, type 2 diabetes mellitus (T2D), PCOs, and other metabolic syndromes. Increasing women's body weight and obesity are the main factors in the pathogenesis of PCOS. It is also associated with endometrial carcinoma, hyperinsulinemia, and insulin resistance. PCO is a good example of a metabolic disorder, which also includes insulin resistance and cardiometabolic risk (**Figure 4**).

Earlier studies reported that women being overweight is the reason for PCOs [61–63]. Conversely, weight loss reduces the risk of reproductive failure, metabolic features of PCOs, and hyperandrogenism [64, 65]. It indicates that treating obesity is the first step to preventing infertility and PCO. Currently, pharmaceutical treatments for obesity are available; however, due to security reasons, there are various limits [66, 67]. Acupuncture treatment is an alternative intervention method for obesity [68]. Some studies suggest that EAT is more effective compared to manual acupuncture, but the effective frequency determination is controversial. In some obesity cases, a combination of diet modification, or exercise, and EAT is essential for weight loss [69, 70].

10.5 Mechanisms of acupuncture treatment on obesity linked PCO

Acupuncture therapy is believed to regulate the hypothalamic–pituitary axis and neuroendocrine. It modulates energy metabolism and eating habits, gastrointestinal

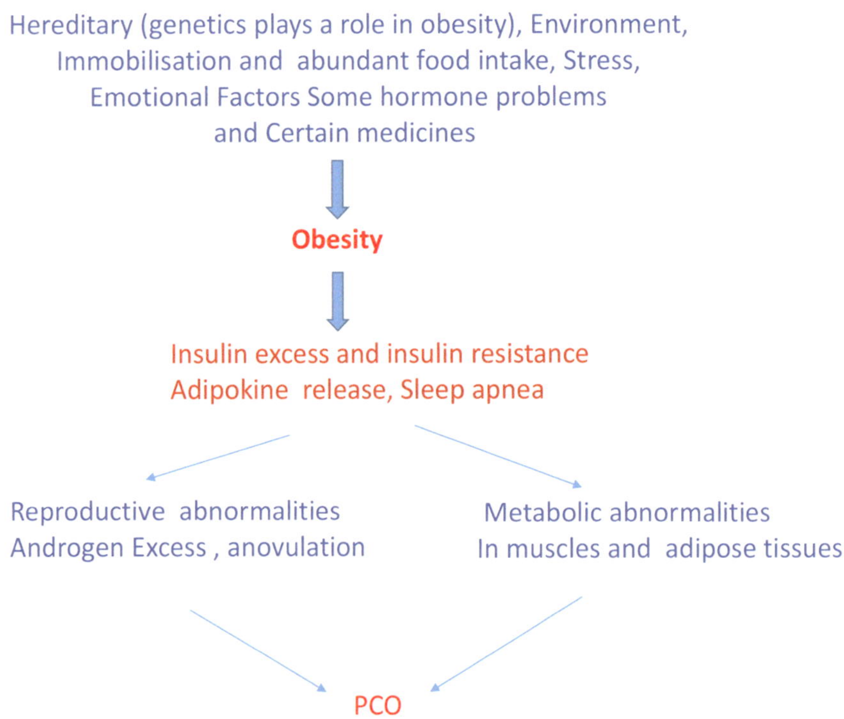

Figure 4.
Summary of obesity linked with PCOS.

tract (GIT) secretions, GI hormones and classic hormones secretions, and nervous system functions [71]. The hypothalamus arcuate nucleus (ARC) contains two microcircuits, agouti-related peptide (AgRP) and neuropeptide-(NPY), which are important for energy balance and have an antagonistic role'. Its signals to stimulate hunger and food intake, and the POMC (pro-opiomelanocortin) signals reduce food intake and satiety. ARC is involved in the central regulation of body weight, energy expenditure, and selected food intake, stimulation of this area alters food intake [72]. Animal model study reveals that EAT reduces food intake; and weight loss and increases the peptide α-MSH and mRNA expression in ARH. Furthermore, EAT significantly reduces the energy intake and body weight in 14-week high-fat diet-fed rats and upregulates the amphetamine-regulated transcript (CART) and cocaine in ARC. It indicates that the valuable effects of EAT act through ARC [73, 74].

Furthermore, specially obesity-linked areas are the Satiety center" in the ventromedial hypothalamus (VMH) and "the feeding center" in the lateral hypothalamus (LH) [75]. Stimulation of these LH centers through EA reduces the excitation of LH, and inhibits hyperorexia-obesity and regulates the catecholamine, ATPase, 5-hydroxytryptamine (5HT) levels in LH [76, 77]. In 1999, Su et al. reported that stimulation of the satiety center, tends to prevent obesity. Through EAT stimulation of the VMH center the levels of dopamine (DA), tyrosine (Tyr), and tryptophan (Typ) ratio were elevated, increasing the excitability of VMH [78].

Research studies believe that normal acupuncture or EAT stimulation increases the spontaneous discharges of nerve cells of the paraventricular nucleus (PVN)

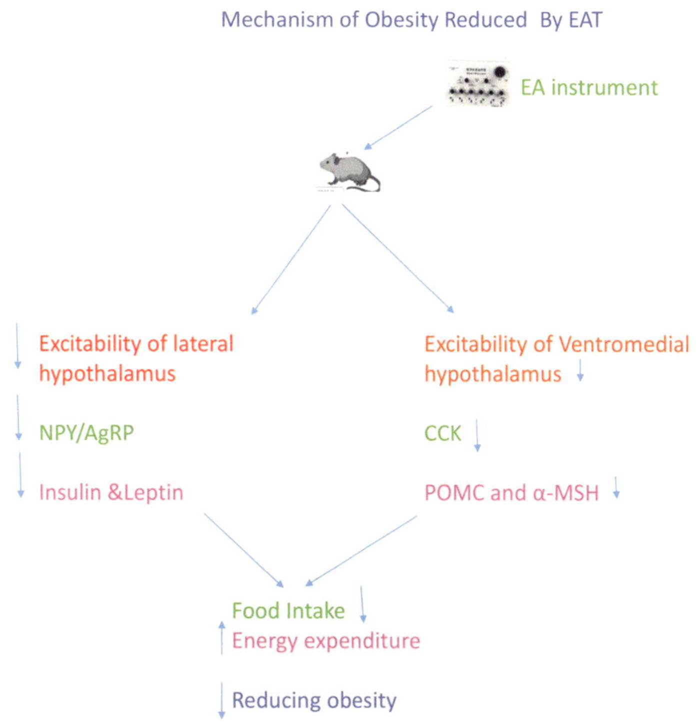

Figure 5.
Neuroendocrine regulation under the effectiveness of acupuncture treatment in the animal model studies. The arcuate nucleus of the hypothalamus (ARH), Ventrosomedial hypothalamus (DMH) lateral hypothalamic area (LHA), paraventricular nucleus (PVN), perifornical nucleus (PeF) Ref [82].

important area for feeding and drinking and decreases the activity of the perifornical nucleus (PeF) The PeF nucleus is important for wakefulness and sleep [79, 80]. Stimulation of the most important acupuncture point in the Stomach 36 (ST36, EA *zusanli*) upregulates the proopiomelanocortin (POMC) in neurons of the Nucleus *Tractus solitarius* (NTS) and hypoglossal nucleus (HN) preventing food intake and leading to weight loss (**Figure 5**) [81].

10.6 Mechanisms of acupuncture treatment on insulin resistance with PCO

Most PCO women are insulin-resistant, particularly obese females [83]. When cells do not respond to insulin, they cannot easily uptake glucose from the blood. It leads to hyperglycemia and excess insulin in the blood (hyperinsulinemia), both of which induce reproductive failure and PCO [84]. Many clinical studies have proved that EAT has beneficial effects on insulin resistance in PCOS patients, and EAT inhibited the insulin resistance of PCO females via activation of the IRS-1/PI3K/GLUT4 pathway [25, 26]. In 2020, Peng Y et al. [7]. reported that in a PCO rat model study, EAT activates the AMPK pathway to suppress SREBP-1 expression, ultimately, inactivating insulin resistance, oxidative stress, and mitochondrial dysfunction (**Figure 6**).

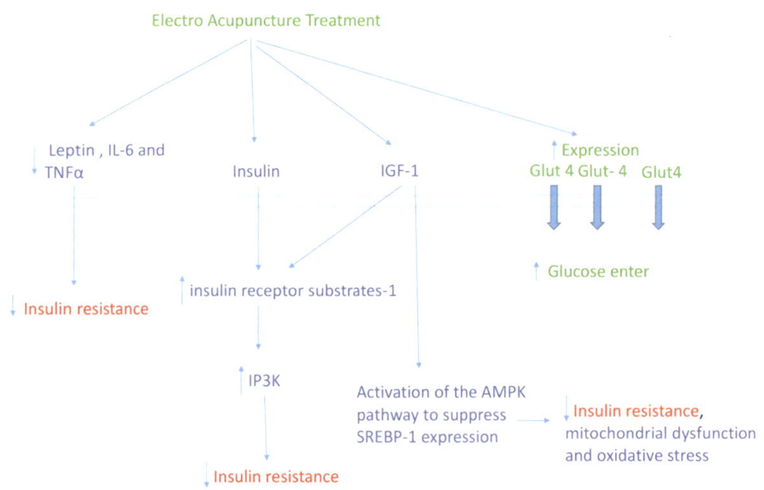

Figure 6.
The effects of EAT on the insulin pathway. EAT upregulates the insulin receptor substrates-1/PI3K/GLUT4 pathway and increases the GLUT4 expression or triggers the adenosine monophosphate-activated protein kinase (AMPK) pathway or stops the PI3K/AKT/mTOR pathway. It also decreases the levels of tumor necrosis factor-α and interleukin-6 both are involved in insulin resistance Ye et al. [85].

The present book chapter summarizes various clinical studies of women with PCOs and PCO animal model studies. Further, it explains the mechanisms of acupuncture and EAT on PCOS-related key symptoms of hyperandrogenism, insulin resistance, ovulatory dysfunction, obesity, and negative emotion. Further, the main acupoints were used for treating women with PCOS, and animals were also described in this chapter.

DOI: http://dx.doi.org/10.5772/intechopen.113799

Author details

Gunasekaran Ramanathan[1,2]

1 Department of Physiology, Swamy Vivekanandha Medical College Hospital and Research Institute, Thiruchangode, TN, India

2 The Tamilnadu Dr. MGR Medical University, Chennai, India

*Address all correspondence to: gunasekaranrr@gmail.com

References

[1] Vos T, Flaxman AD, Naghavi M, Lozano R, Michaud C, Ezzati M, et al. Years lived with disability (YLDs) for 1160 sequelae of 289 diseases and injuries 1990-2010: A systematic analysis for the global burden of disease study 2010. Lancet. 2012;**380**(9859):2163-2196

[2] Escobar-Morreale HF. Polycystic ovary syndrome: Definition, aetiology, diagnosis and treatment. Nature Reviews. Endocrinology. 2018;**14**:270-284

[3] Zhang J, Xin X, Zhang H, Zhu Y, Ye Y, Li D. The efficacy of Chinese herbal medicine in animal models of polycystic ovary syndrome: A systematic review and meta-analysis. Evidence-based Complementary and Alternative Medicine. 2022;**2022**:4892215

[4] Chen Z, Liu L, Xi X, Burn M, Karakaya C, Kallen AN. Aberrant H19 expression disrupts ovarian Cyp17 and testosterone production and is associated with polycystic ovary syndrome in women. Reproductive Sciences. 2022;**29**:1357-1367

[5] Palomba S, Piltonen TT, Giudice LC. Endometrial function in women with polycystic ovary syndrome: A comprehensive review. Human Reproduction Update. 2021;**27**:584-618

[6] Calcaterra V, Verduci E, Cena H, Magenes VC, Todisco CF, Tenuta E, et al. Polycystic ovary syndrome in insulin-resistant adolescents with obesity: The role of nutrition therapy and food supplements as a strategy to protect fertility. Nutrients. 2021;**13**:1848

[7] Peng Y, Guo L, Gu A, Shi B, Ren Y, Cong J, et al. Electroacupuncture alleviates polycystic ovary syndrome-like symptoms through improving insulin resistance, mitochondrial dysfunction, and endoplasmic reticulum stress *via* enhancing autophagy in rats. Molecular Medicine. 2020;**26**:73

[8] Bednarska S, Siejka A. The pathogenesis and treatment of polycystic ovary syndrome: What's new? Advances in Clinical and Experimental Medicine. 2017;**26**:359-367. DOI: 10.17219/acem/59380

[9] Liu H-Y, Liu J-Q, Mai Z-X, Zeng Y-T. A subpathway-based method of drug reposition for polycystic ovary syndrome. Reproductive Sciences. 2014;**22**:423-430

[10] Li Y, Zheng Q, Sun D, Cui X, Chen S, Bulbul A, et al. Dehydroepiandrosterone stimulates inflammation and impairs ovarian functions of polycystic ovary syndrome. Journal of Cellular Physiology. 2018;**234**:7435-7447. DOI: 10.1002/jcp.27501

[11] Vaklavas C, Roberts BS, Varley KE, Lin NU, Liu MC, Rugo HS, et al. TBCRC 002: A phase II, randomized, open-label trial of preoperative letrozole with or without bevacizumab in postmenopausal women with newly diagnosed stage 2/3 hormone receptor-positive and HER2-negative breast cancer. Breast Cancer Research. 2020;**22**:22

[12] Wang R, Li W, Bordewijk EM, Legro RS, Zhang H, Wu X, et al. First-line ovulation induction for polycystic ovary syndrome: An individual participant data meta-analysis. Human Reproduction Update. 2019;**25**:717-732

[13] Balen AH, Morley LC, Misso M, Franks S, Legro RS, Wijeyaratne CN, et al. The management of anovulatory infertility in women with polycystic

ovary syndrome: An analysis of the evidence to support the development of global WHO guidance. Human Reproduction Update. 2016;**22**:687-708

[14] Jia L-Y, Feng J-X, Li J-L, Liu F-Y, Xie L-Z, Luo S-J, et al. The complementary and alternative medicine for polycystic ovary syndrome: A review of clinical application and mechanism. Evidence-Based Complementary Alternatve Medicine. 2021;**2021**:1-12

[15] Rudnicka E, Suchta K, Grymowicz M, Calik-Ksepka A, Smolarczyk K, Duszewska A, et al. Chronic low grade inflammation in pathogenesis of PCOS. International Journal of Molecular Sciences. 2021;**22**:3789. DOI: 10.3390/ijms22073789

[16] Lu L, Zhang Y, Tang X, Ge S, Wen H, Zeng J, et al. Evidence on acupuncture therapies is underused in clinical practice and health policy. BMJ. 2022;**376**:e067475

[17] Zhang B, Shi H, Cao S, Xie L, Ren P, Wang J, et al. Revealing the magic of acupuncture based on biological mechanisms: A literature review. Bioscience Trends. 2022;**16**:73-90

[18] Quiroz-González S, Torres-Castillo S, López-Gómez RE, Jiménez EI. Acupuncture points and their relationship with multireceptive fields of neurons. Journal of Acupuncture Meridian Studies. Apr 2017;**10**(2):81-89

[19] Vickers AJ, Vertosick EA, Lewith G, MacPherson H, Foster NE, Sherman KJ, et al. Acupuncture for chronic pain: update of an individual patient data meta-analysis. Journal of Pain. 2018;**19**(5):455-474

[20] Kong J, Ma L, Gollub RL, Wei J, Yang X, Li D, et al. A pilot study of functional magnetic resonance imaging of the brain during manual and Electroacupuncture stimulation of acupuncture point (LI-4 Hegu) in Normal subjects reveals differential brain activation between methods the. Journal of Alternative and Complementary Medicine. 2004;**8**(4)

[21] Dhond RP, Kettner N, Napadow V. Neuroimaging acupuncture effects in the human brain. Journal of Alternative and Complementary Medicine. 2007;**13**(6):603-616

[22] Bianchi M, Jotti E, Sacerdote P, Panerai AE. Traditional acupuncture increases the content of beta-endorphin in immune cells and influences mitogen induced proliferation. American Journal of China Medicine. 1991;**19**:101-104

[23] Wu J, Chen D, Liu N. Effectiveness of acupuncture in polycystic ovary syndrome: A systematic review and meta-analysis of randomized controlled trials. Medicine (Baltimore). 2020;**99**:e20441

[24] Kokosar M, Benrick A, Perfilyev A, Nilsson E, Kallman T, Ohlsson C, et al. A single bout of electroacupuncture remodels epigenetic and transcriptional changes in adipose tissue in polycystic ovary syndrome. Scientific Reports. 2018;**8**:1878

[25] Li J, Wu W, Stener-Victorin E, Ng EHY, Li RHW, Li M, et al. A prospective pilot study of the effect of acupuncture on insulin sensitivity in women with polycystic ovary syndrome and insulin resistance. Acupuncture in Medicine. 2020;**38**:310-318

[26] Xiang S, Xia MF, Song JY, Liu DQ, Lian F. Effect of electro-acupuncture on expression of IRS-1/PI3K/GLUT4 pathway in ovarian granulosa cells of infertile patients with polycystic ovary syndrome-insulin resistance of

phlegm-dampness syndrome. Chinese Journal of Integrative Medicine. 2021;**27**:330-335

[27] Pan W, Li FX, Wang Q, Huang ZQ, Yan YM, Zhao L, et al. A randomized sham-controlled trial of manual acupuncture for infertile women with polycystic ovary syndrome. Integrative Medical Research. 2022;**11**:100830

[28] Johansson J, Redman L, Veldhuis PP, Sazonova A, Labrie F, Holm G, et al. Acupuncture for ovulation induction in polycystic ovary syndrome: A randomized controlled trial. American Journal of Physiology. Endocrinology and Metabolism. 2013;**304**(9):E934-E943

[29] Zheng YH, Wang XH, Lai MH, Yao H, Liu H, Ma HX. Effectiveness of abdominal acupuncture for patients with obesity-type polycystic ovary syndrome: A randomized controlled trial. Journal of Alternative and Complementary Medicine. 2013;**19**(9):740-745

[30] Li Y, Zhang L, Gao J, Yan J, Feng X, He X, et al. Effect of acupuncture on polycystic ovary syndrome in animal models: A systematic review. Evidence-based Complementary and Alternative Medicine. 2021;**2021**:5595478

[31] Stener-Victorin E, Holm G, Janson PO, Gustafson D, Waern M. Acupuncture and physical exercise for affective symptoms and health-related quality of life in polycystic ovary syndrome: Secondary analysis from a randomized controlled trial. BMC Complementary and Alternative Medicine. 2013;**13**:131

[32] Maliqueo M, Benrick A, Alvi A, Johansson J, Sun M, Labrie F, et al. Circulating gonadotropins and ovarian adiponectin system are modulated by acupuncture independently of sex steroid or beta-adrenergic action in a female hyperandrogenic rat model of polycystic ovary syndrome. Molecular and Cellular Endocrinology. 2015;**412**:159

[33] Jedel E, Labrie F, Oden A, Holm G, Nilsson L, Janson PO, et al. Impact of electro-acupuncture and physical exercise on hyperandrogenism and oligo/amenorrhea in women with polycystic ovary syndrome: A randomized controlled trial. American Journal of Physiology. Endocrinology and Metabolism. 2011a;**300**(1):E37-E45

[34] Lim DC, Chen W, Cheng LN, Xue CC, Wong FW, O'Sullivan AJ, et al. Acupuncture for polycystic ovarian syndrome. Cochrane Database of Systematic Reviews. 2011;**8**:CD007689

[35] Chen J, Feng S, Zeng J, Wu X, Yang M, Tang H, et al. Effectiveness of electroacupuncture for polycystic ovary syndrome: Study protocol for a randomized controlled trial. Trials. 2016;**17**(1):256

[36] Ramadoss M, Ramanathan G. Effect of electroacupuncture on anovulation, epinephrine and norepinephrine levels in drug induced polycystic ovary rats. International Journal of Science and Research (IJSR). 2017;**6**(1)

[37] Stener-Victorin E, Lundeberg T, Waldenstrom U, et al. Effects of electro-acupuncture on nerve growth factor and ovarian morphology in rats with experimentally induced polycystic ovaries. Biology of Reproduction. 2000;**63**(5):1497-1503

[38] Brawer JR, Munoz M, Farookhi R. Development of the polycystic ovarian condition (PCO) in the estradiol valerate treated rat. Biology of Reproduction. 1986;**35**(3):647-655

[39] Dumesic DA, Hoyos LR, Chazenbalk GD, Naik R,

Padmanabhan V, Abbott DH. Mechanisms of intergenerational transmission of polycystic ovary syndrome. Reproduction. 2020;**159**:R1-R13

[40] Budihastuti UR, Melinawati E, Sulistyowati S, Nurwati I. Electro-acupuncture effect on polycystic ovary syndrome to improve oocytes' growth. Medical Acupuncture. 2019;**31**:379-383

[41] Rashidi BH, Tehrani ES, Hamedani NA, Pirzadeh L. Effects of acupuncture on the outcome of *in vitro* fertilisation and intracytoplasmic sperm injection in women with polycystic ovarian syndrome. Acupuncture in Medicine. 2013;**31**:151-156. DOI: 10.1136/acupmed-2012-010198

[42] Chen X, Tang H, Liang Y, Wu P, Xie L, Ding Y, et al. Acupuncture regulates the autophagy of ovarian granulosa cells in polycystic ovarian syndrome ovulation disorder by inhibiting the PI3K/AKT/mTOR pathway through LncMEG3. Biomedicine & Pharmacotherapy. 2021;**144**:112288

[43] Shi Y, Li L, Zhou J, Sun J, Chen L, Zhao J, et al. Efficacy of electroacupuncture in regulating the imbalance of AMH and FSH to improve follicle development and hyperandrogenism in PCOS rats. Biomedicine & Pharmacotherapy. 2019;**113**:108687

[44] Tong X, Liu Y, Xu X, Shi J, Hu W, Ma T, et al. Ovarian innervation coupling with vascularity: The role of electro-acupuncture in follicular maturation in a rat model of polycystic ovary syndrome. Frontiers in Physiology. 2020;**11**:474

[45] Krishnan A, Muthusami S. Hormonal alterations in PCOS and its influence on bone metabolism. The Journal of Endocrinology. 2017;**232**:R99-R113

[46] Wang Z, Yang L, Dong H, Dong H, Cheng L, Yi P, et al. Effect of electroacupuncture on the kisspeptin system in a pubertal rat model of polycystic ovary syndrome. Acupuncture in Medicine. 2021;**39**:491-500

[47] Ramadoss M, Ramanathan G, Subbiah AJ, Natrajan C. Heart rate changes in electroacupuncture treated polycystic ovary in rats. Journal of Clinical and Diagnostic Research. 2016;**10**(3):CF01-3

[48] Task Force of the European Society of Cardiology and the North American Society of Pacing and Electrophysiology. Heart rate variability: Standards of measurement, physiological interpretation and clinical use. Circulation. 1996;**93**(5):1043-1065

[49] Lara HE, Dissen GA, Leyton V, Paredes A, Fuenzalida H, Fiedler JL, et al. An increased intraovarian synthesis of nerve growth factor and its low affinity receptor is a principal component of steroid-induced polycystic ovary in the rat. Endocrinology. 2000;**141**(3):1059-1072

[50] Chintala KK, Krishna BH, N MR. Heart rate variability in overweight health care students: Correlation with visceral fat. Journal of Clinical and Diagnostic Research. 2015;**9**(1):CC06-CC08

[51] Schmidt J, Landin-Wilhelmsen K, Brännström M, Dahlgren E. Cardiovascular disease and risk factors in PCOS women of postmenopausal age: A 21-year controlled follow-up study. The Journal of Clinical Endocrinology and Metabolism. 2011;**96**(12):3794-3803

[52] Stener-Victorin E, Jedel E, Janson PO, Sverrisdottir YB. Low-frequency electroacupuncture and physical exercise decrease high muscle sympathetic nerve activity in

polycystic ovary syndrome. American Journal of Physiology. Regulatory, Integrative and Comparative Physiology. 2009;**297**(2):R387-R395

[53] Stener-Victorin E, Lundeberg T, Cajander S, et al. Steroid-induced polycystic ovaries in rats: Effect of electro-acupuncture on concentrations of endothelin-1 and nerve growth factor (NGF), and expression of NGF mRNA in the ovaries, the adrenal glands, and the central nervous system. Reproductive Biology and Endocrinology. 2003;**1**:33

[54] Mannerås L, Cajander S, Lönn M, Stener-Victorin E. Acupuncture and exercise restore adipose tissue expression of sympathetic markers and improve ovarian morphology in rats with dihydrotestosterone-induced PCOS. American Journal of Physiology. 2009;**296**(4):R1124-R1131

[55] Manni L, Lundeberg T, Holmäng A, Aloe L, Stener-Victorin E. Effect of electro-acupuncture on ovarian expression of $\alpha(1)$- and $\beta(2)$-adrenoceptors, and p75 neurotrophin receptors in rats with steroid-induced polycystic ovaries. Reproductive Biology and Endocrinology. 2005;**3**:article 21

[56] Stener-Victorin E, Deng Q. Epigenetic inheritance of polycystic ovary syndrome – challenges and opportunities for treatment. Nature Reviews. Endocrinology. 2021;**17**:521-533

[57] Feng Y, Johansson J, Shao R, Manneras-Holm L, Billig H, Stener-Victorin E. Electrical and manual acupuncture stimulation affect oestrous cyclicity and neuroendocrine function in an 5alpha-dihydrotestosterone-induced rat polycystic ovary syndrome model. Experimental Physiology. 2012;**97**:651-662

[58] Zhao QY, Sun Y, Zhou J, Gao YL, Ma GZ, Hu ZH, et al. Effectiveness of herb-partitioned moxibustion combined with electroacupuncture on polycystic ovary syndrome in patients with symptom pattern of kidney deficiency and phlegm-dampne. Journal of Traditional Chinese Medicine. 2021;**41**:985-993

[59] Sun J, Jin C, Wu H, Zhao J, Cui Y, Liu H, et al. Effects of electro-acupuncture on ovarian P450arom, P450c17alpha and mRNA expression induced by letrozole in PCOS rats. PLoS One. 2013;**8**:e79382

[60] Xu G, Zhang A, Liu J, Wang X, Feng J, Chen Y. Effects of electroacupuncture on ovarian expression of the androgen receptor and connexin 43 in rats with letrozole-induced polycystic ovaries. Evidence-based Complementary and Alternative Medicine. 2020;**2020**:3608062

[61] Balen AH, Conway GS, Kaltsas G, et al. Polycystic ovary syndrome: The spectrum of the disorder in 1741 patients. Human Reproduction. 1995;**10**:2107-2111

[62] Barber TM, McCarthy MI, Wass JA, Franks S. Obesity and polycystic ovary syndrome. Clinical Endocrinology. 2006;**65**:137-145

[63] Legro RS. The genetics of obesity. Lessons for polycystic ovary syndrome. Annals of the New York Academy of Sciences. 2000;**900**:193-202

[64] Kiddy DS, Hamilton-Fairley D, Bush A, et al. Improvement in endocrine and ovarian function during dietary treatment of obese women with polycystic ovary syndrome. Clinical Endocrinology. 1992;**36**:105-111

[65] Holte J, Bergh T, Berne C, Wide L, Lithell H. Restored insulin sensitivity but persistently increased early insulin secretion after weight loss in obese women with polycystic ovary syndrome. The Journal of Clinical Endocrinology and Metabolism. 1995;**80**:2586-2593

[66] The Cooperative Group Will Be Evaluated after the Listing of Sibutramine Center. Clinical curative effect and safety research in treatment of the simple obesity with sibutramine hydrochloride capsule. Chinese Journal of Clinical Pharmacy. 2004;**15**:17-20

[67] Wu XK, Stener-Victorin E, Kuang HY, et al. Effect of acupuncture and clomiphene in Chinese women with polycystic ovary syndrome: A randomized clinical trial. Journal of the American Medical Association. 2017;**317**(24):2502-2514

[68] Liu Z, Yan S, Wu J, et al. Acupuncture for chronic severe functional constipation: A randomized trial. Annals of Internal Medicine. 2016;**165**(11):761-769

[69] Richards D, Marley J. Stimulation of auricular acupuncture points in weight loss. Australian Family Physician. 1998;**27**(Suppl 2):S73-S77

[70] Mannerås L, Jonsdottir IH, Holmäng A, et al. Low-frequency electroacupuncture and physical exercise improve metabolic disturbances and modulate gene expression in adipose tissue in rats with dihydrotestosterone-induced polycystic ovary syndrome. Endocrinology. 2008;**149**:3559-3568

[71] Hwang SC, Wong EK, Son Y, et al. Neural substrates, experimental evidence, and functional hypothesis of acupuncture mechanisms. Acta Neurologica Scandinavica. 2006;**113**(6):370-377

[72] Joly-Amado A, Cansell C, Denis RG, Delbes AS, Castel J, Martinez S, et al. The hypothalamic arcuate nucleus and the control of peripheral substrates. Best Practice & Research. Clinical Endocrinology & Metabolism. 2014;**28**(5):725-737

[73] Wang F, Tian DR, Tso P, Han JS. Arcuate nucleus of hypothalamus is involved in mediating the satiety effect of electroacupuncture in obese rats. Peptides. 2011;**32**(12):2394-2399

[74] Tian D-R, Li X-D, Wang F, et al. Up-regulation of the expression of cocaine and amphetamine-regulated transcript peptide by electroacupuncture in the arcuate nucleus of diet-induced obese rats. Neuroscience Letters. 2005;**383**(1-2):17-21

[75] Elmquist JK, Elias CF, Saper CB. From lesions to leptin: Hypothalamic control of food intake and body weight. Neuron. 1999;**22**:221-232

[76] Liu ZC, Sun MF, Han Y, et al. Effect of acupuncture on level of monoamines and activity of adenosine triphosphatase in lateral hypothalamic area og obese rats. Chinese Journal of Integrated Traditional and Western Medicine. 2000;**7**:521-523

[77] Zhao M et al. Effect of acupuncture on feeding center of hypothalamus in experimental fat rats. Chinese Acupuncture & Moxibustion. 2001;**5**:49-51

[78] Liu ZC, Sun FM, Su J, et al. Study on action of acupuncture on ventromedial nucleus of hypothalamus in obese rats. Journal of Traditional Chinese Medicine. 2001;**3**:220-224

[79] Liu ZC, Sun MF, Zhao M, et al. Effect of acupuncture on paraventricular nucleus of obese rats. Journal of Traditional Chinese Medicine. 2003;**7**:1031-1033, 1059

[80] Sun Z, Zhang ZC, Ma L, Liu ZC. Effect of acupuncture on expression of hypothalamic neuropeptide Y gene in obese rats. Chinese Journal of Tissue Engineering Research. 2006;**15**:135-138

[81] Ji B, Hu J, Ma S. Effects of electroacupuncture Zusanli (ST36) on

food intake and expression of POMC and TRPV1 through afferents-medulla pathway in obese prone rats. Peptides. 2013;**40**:188-194. DOI: 10.1016/j.peptides.2012.10.009

[82] Zhang K, Zhou S, Wang C, Xu H, Zhang L. Acupuncture on obesity: Clinical evidence and possible neuroendocrine mechanisms. Evidence-based Complementary and Alternative Medicine. 2018;**2018**:6409389

[83] Diamanti-Kandarakis E, Dunaif A. Insulin resistance and the polycystic ovary syndrome revisited: An update on mechanisms and implications. Endocrine Reviews. 2012;**33**:981-1030

[84] Moghetti P, Tosi F. Insulin resistance and PCOS: Chicken or egg? Journal of Endocrinological Investigation. 2021;**44**:233-244

[85] Ye Y, Zhou CC, Hu HQ, Fukuzawa I, Zhang HL. Underlying mechanisms of acupuncture therapy on polycystic ovary syndrome: Evidences from animal and clinical studies. Frontiers in Endocrinology (Lausanne). 2022;**13**:1035929

Chapter 6

Myo-Inositol (ProFecund Ino) – Obtaining a Pregnancy in Women with Polycystic Ovary Syndrome

Isam Al Jashi, Claudia Mehedintu, Miruna Tanase, Mihaela Plotogea, Bogdan Morosan, Edu Antoine and Cristina Gladys Al Jashi

Abstract

Polycystic ovary syndrome (PCOS), affecting 5–10% of women, is characterized by irregular ovulation and excess androgen hormones. The multifactorial causes include hormonal imbalances, insulin resistance, genetics, and obesity. Diagnosis involves identifying criteria like oligo/anovulation, hyperandrogenism, and micro-polycystic ovarian appearance. Traditional treatments include progesterone-based medication and oral contraceptives. However, fertility-focused treatments such as clomiphene, metformin, purified FSH, or LH are administered for those seeking to restore fertility. This article explores "ProFecund Ino," a myo-inositol-based treatment for PCOS. It touts benefits such as improved hormonal balance, regulated menstrual cycles, stimulated ovulation, enhanced insulin sensitivity, and positive effects on the nervous system. The study involving 200 women with PCOS showed a 38% pregnancy rate with ProFecund Ino and additional pregnancies resulted from ovarian stimulation and IVF procedures. The conclusion underscores the efficacy of myo-inositol-based treatments in conjunction with assisted reproductive techniques, significantly increasing pregnancy chances for women with PCOS.

Keywords: polycystic ovary syndrome (PCOS), myo-inositol, ProFecund Ino, fertility treatment, women's health

1. Introduction

Also known as Stein-Leventhal syndrome or chronic hyperandrogenic anovulation, polycystic ovary syndrome (PCOS) is an endocrinological condition characterized by the absence of ovulation and the presence of excessive amounts of androgenic hormones in the female body.

Clinically, PCOS is manifested by amenorrhea (lack of menstrual cycles) or irregular menstrual cycles, accompanied by obesity and manifestations caused by excess androgen hormones (acne, hirsutism, etc.).

2. Epidemiology

PCOS affects 5–10% of the total female population worldwide and up to 26.7% of the female population of childbearing age (15–44 years) [1].

It is estimated that 70% of women with PCOS are still undiagnosed [2].

PCOS symptoms most frequently occur in girls with recent menses and in women in the premenstrual period (with worsening symptoms, especially pelvic pain).

3. Causes and risk factors

The exact cause is not fully elucidated. However, certain favorable factors can be described:

- Disorders of the metabolism of androgen and estrogen hormones;
- Insulin resistance and hyperinsulinemia;
- The genetic factor;
- Obesity.

4. Signs and symptoms

1. Amenorrhea (absence of menstrual cycles) or irregular menstrual cycles;
2. Clinical signs caused by excess androgen hormones (hirsutism—increased body hair, increased muscle mass, acne, alopecia, hoarseness of voice);
3. Obesity.

5. Diagnosis

According to the Rotterdam Consensus of 2003 still in force, the diagnosis of polycystic ovary syndrome (PCOS) is made in the presence of at least two of the following three criteria:

1. Oligo/Anovulation—consequence of ovulatory dysfunction, they are present in about 75% of patients; the remaining 25%, with rhythmic periods, have subclinical oligo/anovulation confirmed by repeated low progesterone levels on day 21 of the menstrual cycle;
2. Clinical and/or biochemical hyperandrogenism—highlighted by the increased value of free testosterone is found in 60–80% of PCOS patients. Among the clinical signs of hyperandrogenism, hirsutism is considered the most relevant (60% of patients), which is evaluated by the modified Ferriman-Gallwey score (mFG). It can associate acne (15–25%) and androgenetic alopecia (5%);

3. Ovaries with a micropolycystic appearance—the micropolycystic appearance of the ovaries is detected by transvaginal ultrasound in 75% of PCOS patients, consisting of at least one ovary with a volume > 10 cm3 or presenting at least 12 follicles with a diameter between 2 and 9 mm.

6. Treatment

Classic treatment includes progesterone-based medication (Medroxyprogesterone) and oral contraceptives.

In the case of women who want to regain their fertility (with the hope of obtaining a future pregnancy), antiestrogens (clomiphene), metformin, and purified FSH or LH are administered.

7. ProFecund Ino

7.1 Active ingredients per daily dose

- Myo-inositol 4000 mg
- Vitex agnus-castus 40 mg
- QuatrefolicTM 755 mcg (400 mcg folate)
- Vitamin B2 2.8 mg
- *Stevia rebaudiana* and fructose (sweeteners) and lemon flavor.

7.2 Mode of presentation

Box with 30 sachets of 3 g of product.

7.3 Administration method

Two sachets per day.

The recommended courses for obtaining a stable result over time are three months.

7.4 Benefits

- Improving female hormonal balance and maintaining a balanced level of testosterone and estrogen (menstrual cycle disorders, premenstrual syndrome, premenopause, hirsutism, acne) [1];
- Regulation of the menstrual cycle and ovulation [2];
- Stimulation of oocyte maturation and increase in the number of oocytes (after ovarian stimulation) [3];
- Improvement of insulin sensitivity [1];

- Optimum functioning of the nervous system and improvement of the emotional state by facilitating the transmission of nerve impulses and improving the sensitivity of brain receptors to serotonin [4, 5];
- Reduces fatigue and protects cells against oxidative stress [5].

8. Myo-inositol

8.1 Definition

Myo-inositol is a pseudovitamin consisting of nine molecules with a similar structure (isomers), found especially in cereals and citrus fruits.

Usually, the term inositol is used for the stereoisomer myo-inositol.

With a similar structure to glucose, inositol is involved in cell signal transmission.

8.2 Indications

8.2.1 Adjuvant in PCOS

One of the causes of polycystic ovary syndrome is insulin resistance. Myo-inositol contributes to increasing insulin sensitivity and improving the activity of insulin receptors.

Also, it contributes to changing the FSH/LH ratio, lowering the testosterone level, and restoring the normal menstrual cycle.

8.2.2 Pregnancy

In pregnant women carrying fetuses with neural tube defects, low levels of inositol have been observed compared to women with normal pregnancies. Inositol can prevent a wide range of neural tube defects resistant to folic acid supplementation.

8.3 Interactions and adverse effects

This shows a high safety profile for most adults. Among the possible side effects that may occur when taking it are nausea and dizziness, fatigue, or headache.

It is considered safe to be given in hospital to premature babies with ARDS (acute respiratory distress syndrome).

In the case of bipolar affective disorders, it is recommended to avoid the administration of inositol, as it may trigger the worsening of symptoms.

No interactions with other drugs are known to date.

9. Vitex agnus-castus

9.1 Characteristics

- Shrub 2–4 m high
- Fruit of chastity/ monks' pepper/ lambing

- Mediterranean and Asian countries
- Blooms in summer
- Goddess Hera—born under a Vitex tree
- Used by Hippocrates
- Mentioned in Materia Medica (Dioscorides)
- Ancient Greece—female adornment during festivals held in honor of Demeter (god of agriculture, fertility, and marriage)

9.2 Mechanism of action

Vitex agnus-castus is not a hormone. Vitex acts on the hypothalamus and pituitary gland where it improves specific hormone secretion or the transmission of the necessary chemical signals to the ovaries for the release of estrogens and progesterone.

$$\text{Vitex agnus-castus} \rightarrow \uparrow LH \text{ and} \downarrow FSH \rightarrow \text{prepares the body for ovulation.}$$

9.3 Vitex and progesterone

Vitex potentiates the hormones involved in ovulation, also participating in the rebalancing of the hormonal balance:

- is effective in regulating pituitary function;
- normalization of estrogen and progesterone levels.

Vitex is highly effective in maintaining adequate progesterone levels during the luteal (postovulatory) phase, levels necessary for pregnancy.

9.4 Interactions and other side effects

- No known drug-extract interactions have been reported for Vitex in humans

  Careful use is recommended when prescribed among:

  - dopamine agonists;
  - hormone replacement therapy (estroprogestant combinations used in the treatment of menopause) due to the mechanisms of action.

- Side effects associated with Vitex extracts are mild, reversible, and uncommon.
- Gastrointestinal disorders or headaches in less than 2% of patients.

10. Quatrefolic

Whereas folic acid requires three intermediate steps to reach the level of active folate, L-Methylfolate (Quatrefolic) is a metabolized folic acid, which leads to its immediate and complete absorption as biologically active folate.

10.1 Benefits: Increased solubility in water

- QuatrefolicTM—100 times more soluble in water compared to the calcium salt of (6S)5- methyl tetrahydrofolic acid—MetafolinTM.

- The high solubility in water of the product means a complete absorption at the level of intestinal cells, facilitating faster access to blood circulation and improving bioavailability at the level of the body.

- Before ingestion, once dissolved in a liquid (water, tea, etc.), the pH of QuatrefolicTM is protected from hydrolytic degradation, which makes it easy to administer.

10.2 Benefits: Increased bioavailability

- The bioavailability of QuatrefolicTM is visibly increased compared to MetafolinTM and folic acid

10.3 Safety of use

- 2010 – USA: GRAS (Generally recognized as safe)

- "For use as a source of folate in conventional and medical foods"

- 2013 – EUROPE: EFSA Positive Scientific Opinion trend

- "As a source of folate added for nutritional purposes to food"

- 2014 – EUROPE: EFSA Novel Food approval

- "As a source of folate added for nutritional purposes to food supplements"

- 2015 – EUROPE: EFSA Novel Food (Annex II to Directive 2002/46/EC)

- "As a source of folate added for nutritional purposes to food supplements"

10.4 Medical uses of quatrefolic

- preconception (planned pregnancy);

- pregnancy;

- breastfeeding;

- newborns, children or adults with folic acid deficiency;
- macrocytic anemia;
- hyperhomocysteinemia.

11. Vitamin B2 (riboflavin)

It is a water-soluble vitamin with an important role in the proper functioning of the entire human body. Water-soluble vitamins, such as vitamin B2, are transported through the bloodstream, and the amount that is no longer needed is eliminated from the body through urine.

Another important aspect is that people must consume vitamin B2 every day, because the body can only store small amounts, and the reserves of this nutrient are consumed quickly.

11.1 Mechanism of action

It acts as an antioxidant, which controls the presence of harmful free radicals inside our body. Riboflavin is necessary for the production of an antioxidant called glutathione, which acts as a "destroyer" of free radicals and, at the same time, detoxifies the liver.

There are many diseases that can be prevented with the help of an adequate dose of riboflavin. This vitamin is also useful in the treatment of genital conditions:

Helps overall metabolism to convert macronutrients: carbohydrates, lipids, and proteins into energy. It also participates in improving the immune system, helps the body to balance acidity, and is important for hair, nails, and eyes.

11.2 Vitamin B2: deficiency

- Stomatitis, the tongue may become red and sore throat, chapped lips and inflammation in the corners of the mouth may occur;
- Eyes may start to sting, redden, water, and become sensitive to light;
- The symptoms, listed above, not taken into account can lead to blood loss;
- Infants whose mothers are deficient in vitamin B2 or have a diet low in vitamin B2 (less than 1.2 mg per day) during pregnancy have a higher risk of certain birth defects.

11.3 Studies

Numerous clinical studies have shown that riboflavin functions as an antioxidant nutrient, effectively mitigating lipid peroxidation and reducing oxidative reperfusion injury. Additionally, a lack of riboflavin may elevate the susceptibility to specific forms of cancer.

Riboflavin may also have neuroprotective effects in certain neurological conditions (e.g., Parkinson's disease, migraine, and multiple sclerosis) through its role.

Less well known is the fact that vitamin B2 provides growth stimulants for children and helps support healthy vision along with vitamin A.

12. Gonal

12.1 Description

Gonal-F (follitropin alpha) is a human follicle-stimulating hormone (FSH) gonadotropin, which is a glycoprotein hormone produced using recombinant DNA technology.

Follitropin alfa possesses a dimeric structure composed of two glycoproteins, the α- and β-subunits, which are non-covalently linked and not identical. The α-subunit comprises 92 amino acids, while the β-subunit has 111 amino acids. Both their primary and tertiary structures closely resemble those of human follicle-stimulating hormone.

The biological activity of follitropin alfa *in vivo* has been standardized against the initial International Standard for Recombinant Human Follicle-Stimulating Hormone, established in 1995 by the Expert Committee on Biological Standards of the World Health Organization.

It is important to note that Gonal-F does not contain any luteinizing hormone (LH) activity.

Gonal-F is a sterile, freeze-dried powder designed for subcutaneous injection following reconstitution. Each Gonal-F multidose vial is supplied with 600 IU (equivalent to 44 micrograms) or 1200 IU (equivalent to 87 micrograms) of follitropin alfa, which delivers 450 IU (about 33 micrograms) or 1050 IU (around 77 micrograms) of follitropin alfa, respectively. These vials also contain 30 milligrams of sucrose, 1.11 milligrams of dibasic sodium phosphate dihydrate, and 0.45 milligrams of monobasic sodium phosphate monohydrate.

12.2 Indications

Gonal-F is indicated for:

- Inducing ovulation and promoting pregnancy in women with oligo-anovulatory infertility, where infertility arises from functional issues (and not due to primary ovarian failure);

- Stimulating the development of multiple follicles in ovulatory infertile women as a component of assisted reproductive technology treatments;

- Inducing spermatogenesis in infertile men with azoospermia (no measurable sperm in semen) and primary or secondary hypogonadotropic hypogonadism when infertility is not a result of primary testicular failure.

12.3 Mechanism of action

Gonal-F encourages the growth of ovarian follicles in women who do not suffer from primary ovarian failure. To trigger the final maturation of the follicle and induce ovulation when a natural LH surge is absent, human chorionic gonadotropin (hCG) is administered after Gonal-F, but only when patient monitoring reveals that adequate follicular development has occurred.

In men with hypogonadotropic hypogonadism, Gonal-F is effective in stimulating spermatogenesis.

13. Cetrotide

13.1 Description

Cetrotide is a medication employed to prevent premature ovulation, which refers to the premature release of eggs from the ovaries. This medication is typically given to women who are undergoing ovarian stimulation treatment, a fertility procedure aimed at stimulating the ovaries to produce a greater number of eggs.

Cetrotide's active ingredient is cetrorelix.

13.2 Mechanism of action

The active ingredient in Cetrotide, cetrorelix, functions by inhibiting the actions of luteinizing hormone-releasing hormone (LHRH) within the body. LHRH regulates the production and release of another hormone known as luteinizing hormone (LH), which is responsible for initiating the process of ovulation. In the context of fertility treatment, ovarian stimulation is utilized to encourage the ovaries to generate a greater number of eggs. By blocking the effects of LHRH, Cetrotide effectively suppresses the production of LH, thereby preventing premature ovulation. This is important because premature ovulation can result in the release of immature and unsuitable eggs for use in assisted reproductive techniques like *in vitro* fertilization (IVF).

14. Study objective

This study aims to increase the chances of obtaining a pregnancy in women diagnosed with polycystic ovary syndrome.

15. Materials and method

This prospective, interventional study had a duration of 24 months, was conducted between January 2021 and February 2023, and was carried out in four national medical centers in Bucharest:

1. Regina Maria – "Unirea" Medical Center;

2. Emergency Clinical Hospital "Sfantul Pantelimon";

3. CMI "Al Jashi Issam";

4. "Nicolae Malaxa" Clinical Hospital

To this purpose, a group of 200 women (aged between 22 and 36 years old) were included.

16. Inclusion criteria

1. Age between 22 and 36 years old.

2. Female, in a relationship.

3. Women with polycystic ovary syndrome (PCOS).

4. The desire to have children and unprotected sexual intercourse 2–3 times a week.

5. Normal values for the partner's semen analysis.

17. Results and discussions

The number of pregnancies installed versus women included in the study: out of the total number of 200 patients who have finalized the study:

38% (76) got pregnant by the end of it;

76% of the remaining patients (94) continued IVF protocol and managed to obtain a pregnancy;

15% will continue with another IVF procedure.

Our study was based on a batch of 200 patients with the environment of origin as shown below (**Figure 1** and **Table 1**):

Our batch of patients was divided between smokers and non-smokers as shown below (**Figure 2** and **Table 2**):

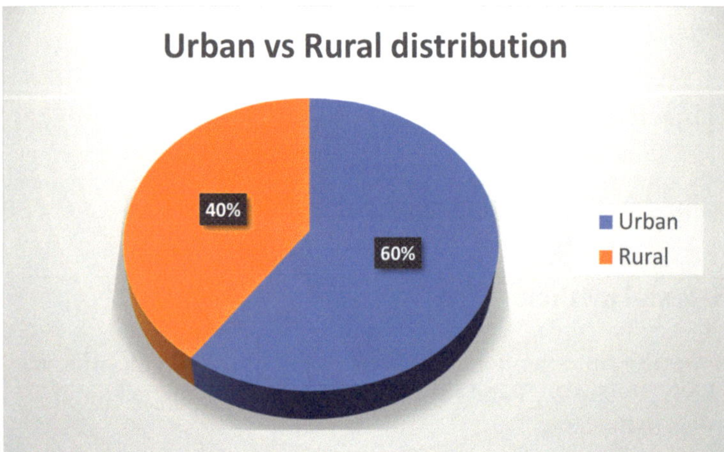

Figure 1.
Patients distribution by living environment.

Total patients 200	
Urban	**Rural**
120	80

Table 1.
Patients distribution by living environment.

The batch presented a small percentage of obese patients (**Figure 3** and **Table 3**):

Out of the 200 women participating in the study, 6% presented comorbidities during their pregnancies. Ten of them presented thrombophilia and two of them gestational diabetes, as shown in **Figure 4** and **Table 4**.

After undergoing between three and six months of ProFecund Ino treatment, 70% of the patients presented follicular quality improvement (**Figure 5** and **Table 5**).

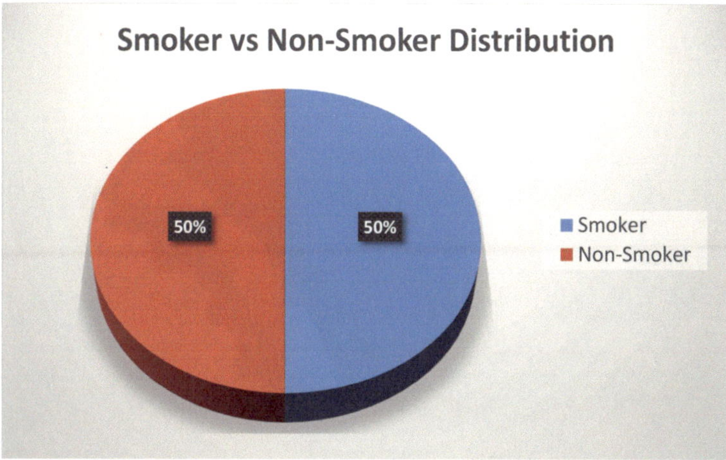

Figure 2.
Smokers vs. nonsmokers distribution.

Total patients 200	
Smokers	**Nonsmokers**
100	100

Table 2.
Smokers vs. nonsmokers distribution.

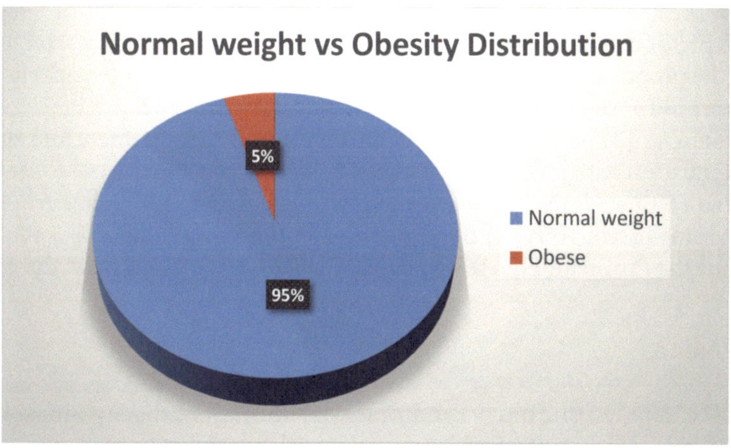

Figure 3.
Normal weight vs. obesity distribution.

Total patients 200	
Normal weight	**Obesity**
190	10

Table 3.
Normal weight vs. obesity distribution.

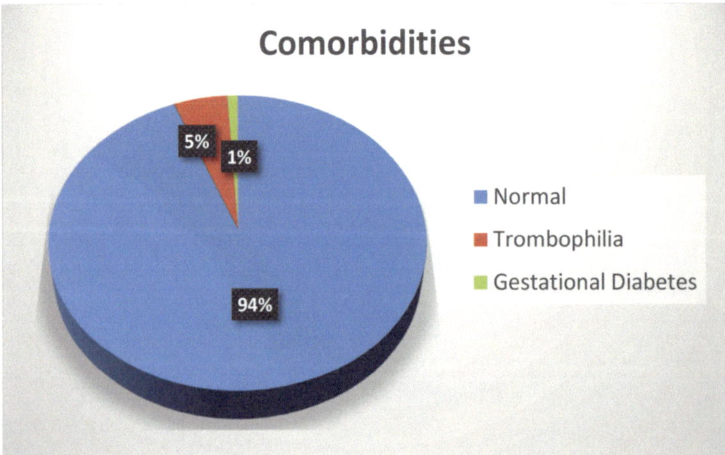

Figure 4.
Comorbidities.

Total patients 200		
Normal	**Thrombophilia**	**Gestational diabetes**
188	10	2

Table 4.
Comorbidities.

In total, 38% out of all included patients (76) obtained pregnancy after only following the proposed treatment with ProFecund Ino. All of the 76 patients were at most 32 years old at the time of pregnancy diagnostic (**Table 6**).

The remaining 124 patients continued the ProFecund Ino treatment and started ovarian stimulation with medium dose Gonal F (Follitropin Alpha) and Cetrotide, followed by an IVF procedure. This led to another 94 pregnancies, which represents 76% of the remaining batch. Thirty of the patients (24%) did not obtain a pregnancy and will continue the ProFecund Ino treatment and will undergo a new procedure (**Table 7**).

18. Conclusions

Patients with polycystic ovary syndrome who underwent the myo-inositol (ProFecund Ino – women, ProFecund B – men with relatively good sperm quality) treatment (both partners for at least four months) managed to obtain a pregnancy in 38% of the cases (**Figures 6** and 7).

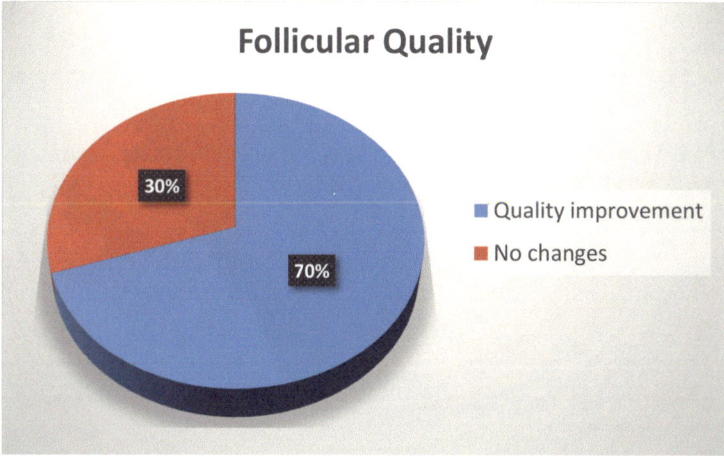

Figure 5.
Follicular quality.

Follicular quality total patients 200	
No changes	**Quality improvement**
60	140

Table 5.
Follicular quality.

Total patients 200	
Pregnancies	**No pregnancy**
76	124

Table 6.
ProFecund Ino ONLY.

Total patients 124	
Pregnancies	**No pregnancy**
94	30

Table 7.
IVF + Profecund Ino.

IVF treatment succeeded in 47% of the total cases after undergoing ProFecund Ino treatment, proceeding with a medium dose of Follitropin Alpha – (Gonal 200 IU) for 7 to 8 days, followed by inhibition with Cetrotide (Cetrorelix) starting on the sixth day of the stimulation process. On the aspiration day, the follicle presented a better quality.

Patients who presented thrombophilia (5%) received antithrombotic treatment with an antiplatelet agent (Aspirin, 75 mg daily) and anticoagulant agent (Clexane,

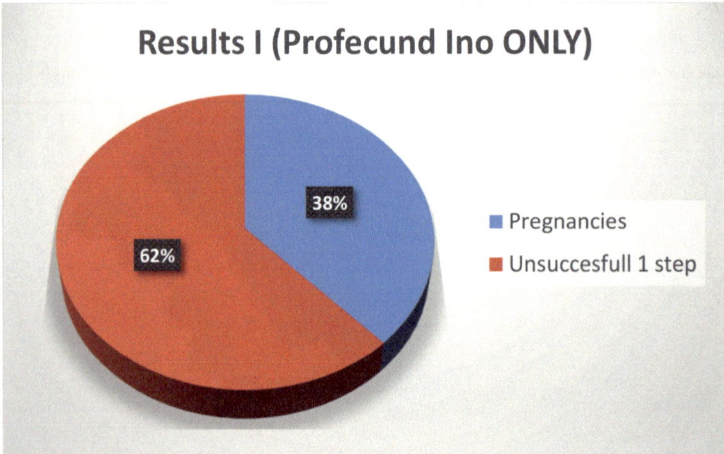

Figure 6.
ProFecund Ino ONLY.

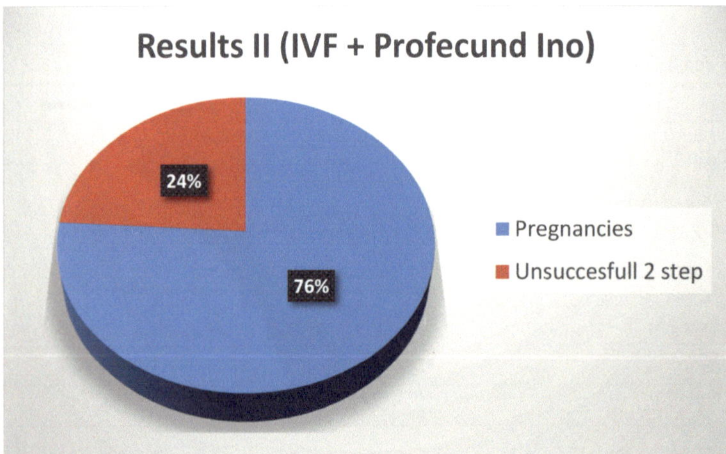

Figure 7.
IVF + ProFecund Ino.

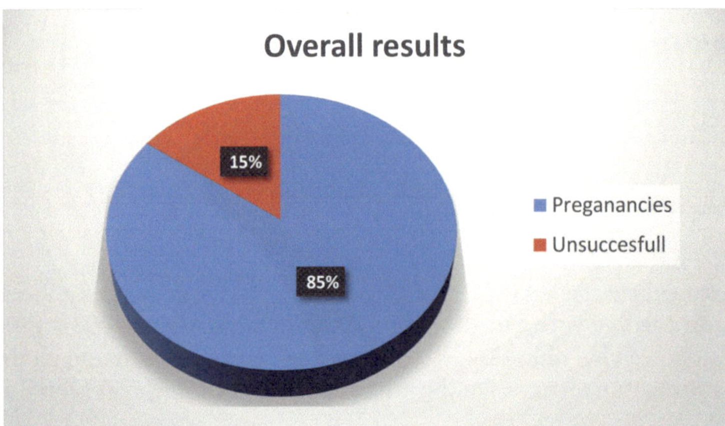

Figure 8.
Overall results.

Total patients 200	
Pregnancies	**Unsuccessful**
170	30

Table 8.
Overall results.

4000UI daily) associated with progesterone. All 10 patients managed to get pregnant and had a full-term delivery.

Patients with gestational diabetes did not necessitate insulin, glucose levels were managed with strict diet.

All patients who carried their pregnancies to term showed an improvement in their polycystic ovary syndrome.

As shown in **Figure 8** and **Table 8**, the main purpose of the study was achieved by obtaining a pregnancy in 85% of the participants and by being able to fulfill their wish of completing their family.

Author details

Isam Al Jashi[1,2], Claudia Mehedintu[3], Miruna Tanase[2], Mihaela Plotogea[4*], Bogdan Morosan[5], Edu Antoine[4] and Cristina Gladys Al Jashi[6]

1 Faculty of Medicine, “Titu Maiorescu” University, Bucharest, Romania

2 Department of Obstetrics and Gynecology, “Unirea Medical Centre” (Regina Maria), Bucharest, Romania

3 Department of Obstetrics and Gynecology, “Filantropia” Clinical Hospital, Bucharest, Romania

4 Department of Obstetrics and Gynecology, “Nicolae Malaxa” Clinical Hospital, Bucharest, Romania

5 Hyllan Pharma, Bucharest, Romania

6 Department of Obstetrics and Gynecology, “Sf. Pantelimon” Emergency Clinical Hospital, Bucharest, Romania

*Address all correspondence to: nicole_plotogea@yahoo.co.uk

References

[1] Unfer V et al. Myo-inositol effects in women with PCOS: A meta-analysis of randomized controlled trials. Endocrine Connections. 2017;**6**(8):647-658. Available from: https://www.ncbi.nlm.nih.gov/pmc/articles/PMC5655679/

[2] Zheng X et al. Inositol supplement improves clinical pregnancy rate in infertile women undergoing ovulation induction for ICSI or IVF-ET. Medicine (Baltimore). 2017;**96**(49):e8842. Available from: https://www.ncbi.nlm.nih.gov/pubmed/29245250

[3] Laganà AS et al. Myo-inositol supplementation reduces the amount of gonadotropins and length of ovarian stimulation in women undergoing IVF: A systematic review and meta-analysis of randomized controlled trials. Archives of Gynecology and Obstetrics. 2018;**298**(4):675-684. Available from: https://www.ncbi.nlm.nih.gov/pubmed/30078122

[4] Palatnik A et al. Double-blind, controlled, crossover trial of inositol versus fluvoxamine for the treatment of panic disorder. Journal of Clinical Psychopharmacology. 2001;**21**(3):335-339. Available from: https://www.ncbi.nlm.nih.gov/pubmed/11386498

[5] Scientific Opinion on the Substantiation of Health Claims related to Riboflavin (vitamin B2). Available from: https://www.efsa.europa.eu/en/efsajournal/pub/1814

Chapter 7

Inositols in the Treatment of Polycystic Ovary Syndrome in Reproductive Age

Neda Smiljan Severinski, Ulla Marton and Anđelka Radojčić Badovinac

Abstract

Polycystic ovary is part of an endocrine syndrome in which different pathophysiological mechanisms lead to a similar reproductive outcome: anovulation, irregularity of the menstrual cycle, and infertility. Hormonal and metabolic disorders are associated with reproductive adverse outcomes, which represent a vicious circle with dysfunctional ovaries. Hyperandrogenemia, disorder of carbohydrate metabolism, and sex hormone synthesis led to reproductive abnormalities. One of the most crucial questions still remains, whether the polycystic ovary is the cause or the consequence of all known disorders. Inositols are in the treatment of PCOS capable of restoring ovulation with the impact on the carbohydrate metabolism, by increasing the sensitivity of cells to insulin, which releases the sex hormones-binding protein and improves hyperandrogenemia. Nine stereoisomers of inositol are known, myo-inositol and chiro-inositol are the most studied in the reproductive age. By normalizing the level of androgens in the blood, the growth of and the balance of sex hormones is established. A variety of metabolic pathways of these molecules are recognized in different tissues, such as fat, muscle, or ovarian tissue. Still, it is not clear which isomer has better reproductive or metabolic effects, and there are controversies about their effectiveness in the treatment of reproductive disorders.

Keywords: D-chiro inositol, inositol, myoinositol, polycystic ovary, pregnancy

1. Introduction

Polycystic ovarian syndrome (PCOS) is defined as a heterogeneous disorder involving a variety of serious clinical manifestations, hormonal disorders, unbalanced metabolic functions, and psychological disorders in women of reproductive age with the main impact on infertility [1]. Rotterdam criteria covered all aspects of this well-acknowledged syndrome with a wide variety of clinical presentations. The four phenotypes of PCOS syndrome are defined, and there is one fundamental criterion—hyperandrogenemia with or without hyperandrogenism in three phenotypes [2]. Evidence suggests the role of different external and internal factors as disorders in the metabolism of carbohydrates with hyperinsulinemia and insulin resistance (IR). Metabolic disorders have an impact on hormonal production, causing serious hormonal dysfunction and disorder that interferes with the dysfunction of ovaries. Polycystic ovary is characterized by a significantly larger content of primordial follicles, therefore enhanced number of granulosis cells that synthesize up to 75 times more anti-Müllerian hormones in granulosa cells of normal ovaries [3]. In women of reproductive age, anovulation, and irregular, extended menstrual cycles are the main causes of infertility. Anovulation is treated primarily by ovulation induction with clomiphene citrate or aromatase inhibitors. Failure of ovarian response in PCO patients on clomiphene induction has introduced gonadotropins as an optional medicamentous treatment to achieve ovulation. The use of gonadotropins includes significant risks of hyperstimulation, thrombo-embolic incidents, or ovarian torsions with possible ovarian necrosis. Niche for the introduction of new promising molecules for therapeutic indications as a useful, effective, and safe tool for restoring spontaneous ovulation has put inositols in focus. Inositols became very interesting and promising molecules due to their biochemical pathways, which are safe in their action and have an effective role in the metabolism of carbohydrates, just like insulin. Inositols are messenger molecules with an impact on enhanced insulin effect in the cells, and specific foods contain them in significant quantities. A positive effect of inositols on ovarian function, ovulation, carbohydrate metabolism, infertility treatment, the incidence of gestational diabetes, and eutrophic newborns after infertility treatment was observed. Inositols improve development of follicules and oocytes, oocyte maturation, fertilization, implantation, and post-implantation development, bringing positive outcomes in IVF procedures in patients with PCOS by reducing the occurrence of gestational diabetes. Reproductive abnormalities are more common in women with higher BMI and continue to rise with higher BMI. Obese women are more likely to have anovulatory cycles and menstrual irregularities. Obesity complicated by metabolic abnormalities can further worsen the outcome of treatment in PCOS patients. Inositols as "messenger" molecules that have a role in insulin signaling with increase effects of insulin intracellularly through phosphoglycan mediators. Naturally, inositols are synthesized mostly in the kidney, with the highest concentration in the brain, where they play a substantial role in neurotransmitters and some steroid hormones binding to their receptors. There are nine isomers of inositol, and differences in the action of these molecules in different tissues, such as fat, muscle, or ovarian tissue, have also been noted. It is not entirely clear which isomer has better reproductive or metabolic effects, and there are controversies and discussions about their effectiveness in the treatment of reproductive disorders, which we will present in this chapter.

2. Metabolic consequences and effect of insulin and inositol

Mechanisms of insulin action and signal transmission to cells of various tissues that use glucose as an energy source are well known. Insulin forms a complex with the insulin receptor that activates phosphatidyl inositol-3 kinase, which is an enzyme that increases the concentration of *phosphoinositides* (PIPs) in cells that integrate molecules into the cell membrane. Four cellular processes are activated in this way: glucose uptake, glycogenesis, antigluconeogenesis, and antilipolysis [4]. Phosphatidyl inositol-3 kinase also activates another messenger of insulin, phosphatidyl inositol, which also stimulates all metabolic activities of insulin and therefore acts synergistically with insulin and enhances its action.

Inositols generally enhance the effects of insulin and regulate intracellular functions: *phosphoinositides* (PIPs)—integrate molecules into the cell membrane *inositol polyphosphates* (InsPs)—are cytoplasmic "second" messengers and *inositol phosphoglycans* (IPGs) regulate mitochondrial metabolism [5]. Inositols are very stable polar molecules that belong to the family of nine *hexahydroxycyclohexane stereoisomers*. They were initially isolated from muscles and later from numerous cells and tissues of mammals. In addition to insulin signal transmission, they are very active in cellular processes such as calcium transport, association of cytoskeletal proteins, lipid metabolism, modulation of the serotoninergic pathway, cell growth and differentiation, and oocyte maturation. Inositol isomers have been proven to have an important role in various medical conditions such as neurodegenerative diseases (scyllo inositol), diabetes (D-chiro inositol, DCI), malignant diseases, metabolic syndrome, or PCO syndrome (myo-inositol, MI).

Myo-inositol is the most widespread molecule among inositols in nature and mammalian cells (99%); the rest is D-chiro inositol (1%). Myo-inositol is converted into DCI by epimerization (the metabolic pathway is stimulated by the tissue-specific NAD/NADH epimerase that is dependent on insulin), which significantly changes the concentration ratio of these molecules in tissues such as the liver, adipose tissue, or muscle, respectively, to the brain. Myo-inositol is found in cells in free form or bound in cell membranes (in the composition of *phosphoinositide*), i.e., it is a protector of hyperosmotic stress in cells. As a second messenger, it regulates the activity of a number of hormones, such as follicle-stimulating hormone (FSH), thyroid-stimulating hormone (TSH), and insulin. In mammals, a tissue-specific epimerase converts MI to DCI in an insulin-dependent manner, and different ratios of these epimers have been confirmed in different tissues. D-chiro inositol is an important molecule in the insulin signaling pathway and, together with galactosamine, significantly affects molecular mechanisms (activation of molecules that alleviate the consequences of glucose metabolism disorders). However, paradoxically in women with IR and pre-eclampsia the concentration of DCI is elevated and it is suspected that DCI contributes to IR [6, 7].

3. Ovary, insulin resistance, and hyperandrogenemia

Ovarian function disorders in PCOS represent a growing heterogeneous, multifaceted complex entity, combined with a metabolic disorder caused by deterioration in the metabolism of carbohydrates and insulin resistance (IR). Insulin resistance is defined as a subnormal biological response to normal insulin levels, decreased sensitivity, or response to metabolic action of insulin. Clinically, insulin resistance can be described as the insufficient cell response of a known quantity of endogenous or exogenous insulin to increase glucose uptake and reduced sensitivity or answer to the metabolic effect of insulin. The significant association of PCO syndrome and IR is seemingly, obvious highly, complex and problematic. The frequency of association between IR and PCO according to the literature, depends on the studied population and different criteria used in the published studies. Although IR is significantly associated with PCO syndrome, it is not established as diagnostic criteria for PCO syndrome. Similarly, there are no general recommendations for screening for IR in patients with PCO syndrome. Obesity is frequently associated with PCO syndrome and plays a key role in hyperinsulinemia and IR. There are debates about interactions and relations of obesity, IR, and PCO syndrome. Accumulation of adipocytes in adipose tissue plays an important role in the endocrine function of the ovary. The enhanced production of leptin in adipocytes inhibits the expression of aromatase mRNA in granulosa cells, causing interruption of androgen conversion to estrogen. Production of adiponectin in adipocytes has insulin-sensitizing, anti-diabetic, and anti-inflammatory effects. It is unclear whether obesity is the cause of IR or worsens already-existing IR in PCO syndrome. Published data indicate that obesity is an additional circumstance that aggravates IR in patients with already previously existing IR [8, 9]. Systemic hyperinsulinism can be endogenous (obesity, gestational diabetes, diabetes type 2, extreme IR caused by mutation of the insulin receptor gene, autoantibodies on insulin receptor, insulinoma) or exogenous (diabetes mellitus type 1). HOMA-IR is a frequent parameter used in estimating IR in large epidemiological population studies and is calculated as a ratio of fasting insulin and glucose values. HOMA-IR can be increased in code-slender or obese patients with PCO syndrome in comparison to patients without PCO syndrome. According to the published results [9], cut-off value of HOMA-IR is 3.15 for patients with PCO syndrome, while in the general population, the defined cut-off value of HOMA-IR is 2.5. The assessment of insulin resistance is one of the major questions for clinicians, remaining how to distinguish wide variability in insulin-sensitive female patients in relation to insulin insensitivity and what criteria are acceptable in different ethnic groups. The fact is that not all women with IR have PCO syndrome, and the same IR is not present in all women with PCO syndrome. Insulin levels depend on several factors, such as metabolism and clearance of insulin, enzymatic degradation of the insulin - receptor complex, obesity, age, and androgen level. It should be taken into concern during the evaluation of the patient. To conclude, there might be some additional factor that leads to hyperandrogenism, which is an obligatory diagnostic criterion included in PCO syndrome and associated with hyperinsulinemia or some additional trigger. Hyperandrogenism has an important impact on the mechanism of PCOS, including IR, inflammation, and oxidative stress. Hyperandrogenism aggravates IR through different routes, by inhibiting insulin degradation in the liver and reduction of insulin sensitivity. Still, we need to define the necessary criterion for the diagnosis of HA as an additional trigger for the development of PCO syndrome with hyperinsulinemia.

Insulin resistance and compensatory hyperinsulinism, contribute to increased production of androgens. Insulin has a modality as gonadotropin in the ovary triggering ovarian steroidogenesis, stimulating androgen synthesis in the adrenal glands, and modulates pulsatility of LH by increasing LH binding sites and androgen-producing response to LH. Hyperandrogenemia is responsible for reproductive disorders like ovulatory dysfunction, anovulation, oligomenorrhea, infertility, acne, and alopecia, which are clinical signs of PCO syndrome. Hyperandogenemia is associated with obesity and increased visceral fat, which are not rare in patients with PCO syndrome. An increase in fat tissue promotes IR, HA, and hyperinsulinemia, and again, we are in the same circle of alternating disorders [1]. The genomic, transcriptomic, and proteomic profile of visceral fatty tissue in women with PCO syndrome is different from that of healthy women, more similar to a man's fatty tissue, and hence suggests the metabolic effect of HA on typical obesity in PCO syndrome [10]. Beyond the multifactorial pathophysiology of PCOS, one of the hypotheses suggests a pathogenetic role of high levels of androgens that are the main cause of abdominal and visceral fatty tissue accumulation. Both stimulate IR and compensatory hyperinsulinism. Hyperinsulinism is responsible for androgen synthesis in the ovary and adrenal glands and promotes leptin-mediated inflammation in women with PCO syndrome, so the vicious circle closes [1]. Heterogeneity of PCO syndrome most likely arises from obesity, abdominal fat, and IR. Central hepatic insulin resistance can be present in slender patients with PCO syndrome, while the peripheral IR is tied to adipose tissue and muscles and is characteristic of female patients who are obese.

Since some inositols (MI, DCI) are mediators of insulin, they can potentially change the metabolism of various tissues. Inositols are credited with acting as a second messenger, in response to external or endocrine signals, reducing IR, improving ovarian function by reducing androgen levels, and alleviating metabolic, menstrual, and cutaneous hyperandrogenic features of PCOS. Noticeably, inositols are involved in the action of several endocrine systems (insulin, thyroid hormone, gonadotropins) and lipids with hormone-like activity signals (as prostaglandins). Myo-inositol and DCI are the two most abundant members of nine stereoisomeric inositols. The specificities of the inositols metabolism in the ovary and differences compared to other tissues are known. D-chiro inositol is synthesized *in vivo* by epimerization from MI, and the degree of epimerization defines insulin-dependent epimerase. The ratio of MI and DCI concentration in ovarian tissues is 70:1, while the ratio in women with PCOS is pathologically decreased. Type 2 diabetes mellitus, with its pathophysiological pathways, can dramatically impair DCI levels, resulting in low intracellular levels of DCI due to reduced activity of epimerase (hyperinsulinemia reduces activity of epimerase). In PCO syndrome, ovaries are in a state in which tissue-selective resistance to metabolic effects of insulin seems to be contradictory and associated with ovarian sensitivity to insulin unlikely liver, fat, and muscle tissue. In PCO syndrome with pronounced hyperinsulinemia, in the ovary, there is an accelerated conversion of MI to DCI (increased ratio, excessive synthesis of DCI) due to accelerated epimerization. As a consequence, deficiency of MI in the ovary causes specific reproductive disturbances [11]. This phenomenon, called the D-chiro inositol paradox, is a rebound effect on hyperinsulinemia. The mechanism involves tissue-specific metabolic pathways that decrease the synthesis of DCI in the liver, muscles, and fat tissue as a response to hyperinsulinemia; under the same circumstances, DCI synthesis increases within the ovaries while synthesis of MI is lacking. Therefore, DCI is effective in treating and reducing IR but not in reducing ovarian disorders in PCO patients [12].

4. Treatment of reproductive disorders with inositols

Reproductive abnormalities in PCO syndrome may appear with different clinical presentations. Disorders of ovulation, oligomenorrhea, amenorrhea, and menstrual cycle irregularities are the most common infertility causes in patients with PCO syndrome [13]. The different clinical PCOS phenotypes require proper assessment of the biochemical and medical features to adopt the best pharmacological treatment and therapeutic strategy in patients with PCO syndrome. The aim of the pharmacological treatment may be hyperandrogenemia, oligo-ovulation, or IR. The therapeutic management and selection of the best therapy should be done upon the clinical features of the target patient and her priorities—regulation of menstrual disturbance, ovulation abnormalities, oligo-ovulation, hyperandrogenism or IR, or altogether. Before drug administration, diet and healthy lifestyle advice must be given to all patients with PCOS regardless of their weight.

Physical activity and exercise (150 min of moderate or 75 min of intense exercise per week) play a key role in weight reduction and the prevention of obesity. That approach has been proven to be the best way to improve insulin sensitivity. Weight reduction with calorie intake restriction and the introduction of physical activity would be the first step in treatment for obese women diagnosed with PCO syndrome. With weight loss, the free testosterone level decreases, as does the incidence of metabolic syndrome. Changes in lifestyle and diet lead to lower insulin and free androgen levels, inducing the restoration of body composition, hyperandrogenism, and IR. There is very much to discover, for a better understanding of pathogenesis, how the reduction of fat tissues modifies all metabolic pathways and improvements in the metabolism of glucose or lipids, reproductive outcome, mood, quality of life, and therapy satisfaction [14]. Weight reduction leads to better self-esteem.

Hyperinsulinemia and IR are key goals of treatment in patients with PCO syndrome and include the administration of insulin-sensitizing drugs (e.g. metformin). There is still no definite cure or medication for this heterogeneous endocrine disorder with various clinical appearances. The routine approach after advising on lifestyle modification and weight loss is symptomatic therapy with different agents including oral antidiabetics, progesterone, contraceptives, or antiandrogens. The efficiency and efficacy of some other drugs as thiazolidinediones, berberine, or inositols have not been enough investigated and the effects of these drugs are still unclear in infertility treatment.

Classic gynecological treatment in reproductive-age patients with PCO syndrome implies regulation of the menstrual cycle with the administration of combined oral hormonal contraception or progestins. Induction of ovulation is required in PCOS patients with anovulatory cycles if there is a desire for motherhood. The first-line treatment for ovulation induction is clomiphene citrate and letrozole, especially if it is a fertility problem tied only to anovulation without co-existing male factor or tubal obstruction. In the cases of combined male–female infertility, couples are treated with assisted reproductive technologies (*in vitro* fertilization) and stimulation of ovaries with gonadotropins. The use of gonadotropins carries significant risks of ovarian hyperstimulation, and that's why they have indicated targeted protocols for ovarian stimulation. From the point of patient safety, treatment with an antagonist for ovarian stimulation and the "freez all" approach are the best options if there is ovarian hyperstimulation. Ovarian stimulation in agonistic protocol in combination with metformin can reduce the risk of hyperstimulation [15]. Some patients are resistant to ovulation inductors due to persistent hyperandrogenemia, hyperestrogenemia, and IR. This abnormality is further worsened in overweight PCOS patients, especially with visceral and abdominal fatty tissues, since SHBG level is reduced due to hyperinsulinemia, and androgen levels are increasing. Since hyperinsulinemia stimulates androgen synthesis in patients with PCO syndrome, the attention of researchers is focused on inositol phosphoglycans as post-receptor mediators or secondary messengers of insulin signals [16].

Administration of MI in patients with PCO syndrome after 12 weeks has a positive effect on the hormonal status of the patients. It has proven a significant reduction in the concentration of LH, PRL, androgens, and of LH/FSH ratio and ratio glucose/insulin. Increased sensitivity to insulin had been observed by reduction of HOMA-IR. In PCO patients treated with *in vitro* fertilization procedure and inositols it has been observed shorter duration of ovarian stimulation and minor total dose of applied gonadotropins. Severe ovarian hyperstimulation syndrome is significantly more often present in patients with PCO syndrome and associated with increased number of antral follicles. The positive effect of MI was observed in improved response to ovarian stimulation. The group of PCOS patients treated with

MI had significantly more large follicles (> 16 mm) on hCG day administration, compared to control group, which had significantly more small follicles (< 12 mm). The application of MI contributes not only to the safety of infertility treatment but also to the better quality of the follicles. The final reproductive outcome, the proportion of conceived pregnancies and births, decreased incidence of gestational diabetes, and giving birth to eutrophic children are also significantly better in MI users [17, 18]. In patients with PCO syndrome, a higher concentration of DCI in the urine (higher elimination) and at the same time a reduced concentration in the plasma was observed compared to healthy eumenorrhoic women, while no such differences were observed for MI. According to the previously published data, MI supplementation improves many ovarian functions, oocyte quality, ovulation, higher chance of conception with better reproductive outcomes, as well as minor total gonadotropin dose during ovarian stimulation. Both stereoisomers MI and DCI additionally improve the regulation of glucose metabolism, lipid metabolism, and clinical signs of hyperandrogenemia [19–21]. Thus, significant dysregulation of inositol metabolism was demonstrated in patients with PCO syndrome, which indicates a connection with hyperinsulinemia and IR.

Already initial studies have proven the significant effectiveness of DCI in reducing lipid biomarkers, increasing insulin sensitivity, reducing androgen levels, and increasing the frequency of ovulation. These effects are mainly related to the positive systemic effect of DCI on the metabolic syndrome, but not to the effect on the ovary [22, 23], while MI has proven direct positive effects on ovarian function at the cellular level. Administration of higher doses of DCI (2.4 g/day), seems to have a negative effect on ovarian function, more significantly in PCO patients who do not have diagnosed IR. The release of a larger amount of DCI-phosphoglycan with hyperinsulinemia stimulates the biosynthesis of testosterone in ovarian theca cells, which increases hyperandrogenemia and leads ovarian follicles to growth arrest, atresia, or even to anovulation [24, 25].

Newer published studies indicate on positive effects of combined preparations which contain both stereoisomers MI and DCI on ovarian function in patients with PCO syndrome treated with *in vitro* fertilization procedures. The analysis of seven factors of oocyte quality has proved the positive impact of the combined administration of MI and DCI on oocyte quality, with preparations that contained a higher concentration of DCI in relation to MI. The known physiological ratio of MI and DCI in the plasma is 40:1 (in the ovary 100:1), but it seems that the effect on cell quality is still more dependent on the concentration of DCI than on the physiological ratio. The effect of these changes on developing embryos after ICSI fertilization remains unclear, as well as the effect on conception [26]. Studies on the preventive effect of inositol on the occurrence of gestational diabetes in the population of patients with PCO syndrome have also been published [27, 28]. The effect of MI and DCI was evaluated in the population of pregnant women diagnosed with gestational diabetes in mono-formulations or in combination. It was found that there is a significant beneficial effect on metabolic factors and reduction of IR in pregnant women diagnosed with gestational diabetes, and according to the results of the study, it has been shown that DCI has a more significant effect than MI [29, 30]. The choice of medical treatment including inositols depends on undelaying endocrinological and metabolic disorders and treatment goals. The applications of inositols showed clinical benefits in almost all outcomes compared to metformin independently and in combination with other forms of treatment for reproductive disorders.

5. Conclusions

Inositols are very interesting and promising molecules with consideration on their role in carbohydrate metabolism and consideration on their impact on cells with increasing effects of insulin intracellulary. They act as "messenger" molecules, increasing the sensitivity of insulin in targeted cells. Inositols have a positive impact on follicle maturation, they can improve the mechanism of dominant follicle selection by a reduction in free androgen levels by increasing aromatase activity and induction of SHBG production. According to literature data, it has been proved that inositol had favorable effect on several results of outcomes in patients with PCO syndrome. Present scientific results proved that inositols have a beneficial impact on ovarian function establishing ovulation, a positive effect on carbohydrate metabolism, on occurrences of gestational diabetes, and giving birth to eutrophic newborns. The positive effects of both stereoisomers MI and DCI as well as their combinations, on metabolic parameters, IR, regulation of glucose metabolism, and reproductive disorders have been scientifically proven. According to the data published so far, DCI has its greatest effectiveness in states with pronounced IR. Myo-inositol, on the other hand, has proven positive direct effects on ovarian function at the cellular level. Replacement of a single isomer, or their combination, is based on different actions and biological roles. The choice of treatment depends on which underlying disorder we want to treat. The clinical application of these substitutes has proven the beneficial effects of these molecules independently and in combination with other forms of treatment for reproductive disorders.

Acknowledgements

The publication is supported by H2020 MESOC–measuring the social dimension of culture; under Grant Agreement no. 870935. Uniri-biomed-18-161project: Extracellular vesicles in human follicular fluid: content and role in oocyte maturation and embryo quality.

Conflict of interest

The authors declare no conflict of interest.

Author details

Neda Smiljan Severinski[1]*, Ulla Marton[2] and Anđelka Radojčić Badovinac[3,4]

1 Faculty of Medicine Rijeka, Department of Gynecology and Obstetrics, Clinical Hospital Center Rijeka, University of Rijeka, Croatia

2 Faculty of Medicine Rijeka, University of Rijeka, Poliklinika "dr. Marton", Zagreb, Croatia

3 Department of Biotechnology, University of Rijeka, Rijeka, Croatia

4 Faculty of Medicine Rijeka, Department of Medical Biology and Genetics, University of Rijeka, Rijeka, Croatia

*Address all correspondence to: nedass@uniri.hr

References

[1] Escobar-Morreale HF. Polycystic ovary syndrome: Definition, aetiology, diagnosis and treatment. Nature Reviews Endocrinology. 2018;**14**(5):271-284

[2] Radojčić Badovinac A, Smiljan Severinski N. Polycistic ovary syndrome phenotypes and infertility treatment. In: Polycistic Ovary Syndrome–Functional Investigation and Clinical Application. London, UK: IntechOpen; 2022. DOI: 10.5772/ontechopen.101994

[3] Pellat L, Hanna L, Brincat M, Galea R, Brain H, Whitehead HM. Granulosa cell production of anti-Müllerian hormone is increased in polycystic ovaries. The Journal of Clinical Endocrinology and Metabolism. 2007;**92**(1):240-245

[4] Yaribeygi H, Farrokhi FR, Butler AE, Sahebkar A. Insulin resistance: Review of the underlying molecular mechanisms. Journal of Cellular Physiology. 2019;**234**(6): 8152-8161

[5] Genazzani AD. Inositol as putative integrative treatment for PCOS. Reproductive Biomedicine Online. 2016;**33**:770-780

[6] Bevilacqua A, Bizzarri M. Physiological role and clinical utility of inositols in polycystic ovary syndrome. Best Practice & Research Clinical Obstetrics & Gynaecology. 2016;**37**:129-139

[7] Croze ML, Soulage CO. Potential role and therapeutic interest of myo-inositol in metabolic diseases. Biochimie. 2013;**95**(10):1811-1827

[8] Teede HJ, Hutchison SK, Zoungas S, Meyer C. The management of insulin resistance in polycystic ovary syndrome. Trends in Endocrinology and Metabolism. 2007;**18**:273-279

[9] Alebic MS, Bulum T, Stojanovic N, Duvnjak L. Definition of insulin resistance using the homeostasis model assessment (HOMA-IR) in IVF patients diagnosed with polycystic ovary syndrome (PCOS) according to the Rotterdam criteria. Endocrine. 2014;**47**:625-630

[10] Montes-Nieto R, Insenser M, Martinez-Garcia MA, Escobar-Morreale HF. A nontargeted proteomic study of the influence of androgen excess on human visceral and subcutaneous adipose tissue proteomes. The Journal of Clinical Endocrinology and Metabolism. 2013;**98**:E576-E585

[11] Matalliotakis I, Kourtis A, Koukoura O, Panidis D. Polycystic ovary syndrome: Etiology and pathogenesis. Archives of Gynecology and Obstetrics. 2006;**274**:187-197

[12] Carlomagno G, Unfer V, Roseff S. The D-chiro-inositol paradox in the ovary. Fertility and Sterility. 2011;**95**(8):2515-2516

[13] Beliver J, Rodriguez-Tabernero L, Robles A, Muňos E, Martinez F, Landeras J, et al. Polycistic ovary syndrome throughout a woman's life. Journal of Assisted Reproduction and Genetics. 2018;**35**(1):225-239

[14] Moran LJ, Hutchison SK, Norman RJ, Teede HJ. Lifestyle changes in women with polycystic ovary syndrome. Cochrane Database of Systematic Reviews. 2011;**2**:CD007506

[15] Balen AH, Morley LC, Misso M, Franks S, Legro RS, Wijeyaratne CN,

et al. The management of anovulatory infertility in women with polycystic ovary syndrome: An analysis of the evidence to support the development of global WHO guidance. Human Reproduction Update. 2016;**22**:687-708

[16] Reyes-Mun˜oz E, Sathyapalan T, Rossetti P, Shah M, Long M, Buscema M, et al. Polycystic ovary syndrome: Implication for drug metabolism on assisted reproductive techniques—a literature review. Advances in Therapy. 2018;**35**:1805-1815. DOI: 10.1007/s12325-018-0810-1

[17] Costantino D, Minozzi G, Minozzi F, Guaraldi C. Metabolic and hormonal effects of myo-inositol in women with polycystic ovary syndrome:A double-blind trial. European Review for Medical and Pharmacological Sciences. 2009;**13**:105-110

[18] Artini PG, Di Berardino OM, Papini F, Genazzani AD, Simi G, Ruggiero M, et al. Endocrine and clinical effects of myo-inositol administration in polycystic ovary syndrome. A randomized study. Gynecological Endocrinology. 2013;**29**(4):375-379. DOI: 10.3109/09513590.2012.743020

[19] Baillargeon JP, Diamanti-Kandarakis E, Ostlund RE, et al. Altered D-chiro-inositol urinary clearance in women with polycystic ovary syndrome. Diabetes Care. 2006;**29**:300-305

[20] Baillargeon JP, Nestler JE, Ostlund RE, Apridonidze T, Diamanti-Kandrakis E. Greek hyperinsulinemic women, with or without polycystic ovary syndrome, display altered inositols metabolism. Human Reproduction. 2008;**23**(6):1439-1446. DOI: 10.1093/humrep/den097

[21] Facchinetti F, Dante G, Neri I. The ratio of MI to DCI and its impact in the treatment of polycystic ovary syndrome: Experimental and literature evidences. In: Genazzani A, Tarlatzis B, editors. Frontiers in Gynecological Endocrinology. ISGE Series. Cham: Springer; 2016. DOI: 10.1007/978-3-319-23865-4_13

[22] Lagana` AS, Barbaro L, Pizzo A. Evaluation of ovarian function and metabolic factors in women affected by polycystic ovary syndrome after treatment with D-chiro-inositol. Archives of Gynecology and Obstetrics. 2015;**291**:1181-1186

[23] Fruzzetti F, Capozzi A, Canu A, Lello S. Treatment with D-chiro-inositol and alpha lipoic acid in the management of polycystic ovary syndrome. Gynecological Endocrinology. 2019;**35**(6):506-510

[24] Rosalbino I, Raffone I. Does ovary need D-chiro-inositol? Journal of Ovarian Research. 2018;**11**(5):57. DOI: 10.1186/1757-2215-5-14

[25] Nestler JE, Jakubowicz DJ, De Vargas AF, Brik C, Quintero N, Medina F. Insulin stimulates testosterone biosynthesis by human thecal cells from women with polycystic ovary syndrome by activating its own receptor and using inositolglycan mediators as the signal transduction system. The Journal of Clinical Endocrinology and Metabolism. 1998;**83**(6):2001-2005. DOI: 10.1210/jc.83.6.2001

[26] Mendoza N, Galan MI, Molina C, Mendoza-Tesarik R, Conde C, Mazheika M, et al. High dose of D-chiro-inositol improves oocyte quality in women with polycystic ovary syndrome undergoing ICSI: A randomized controlled trial. Gynecological Endocrinology. 2020;**36**(5):398-401. DOI: 10.1080/09513590.2019.1681959

[27] Matarrelli B, Vitacolonna E, D'angelo M, Pavone G, Mattei PA, Liberati M,

et al. Effect of dietary myo-inositol supplementation in pregnancy on the incidence of maternal gestational diabetes mellitus and fetal outcomes: A randomized controlled trial. The Journal of Maternal-Fetal & Neonatal Medicine. 2013:**26**(10):967-972. DOI: 10.3109/14767058.2013.766691. Epub 2013 Mar 1. PMID: 23327487

[28] Farren M, Daly N, McKeating A, Kinsley B, Turner MJ, Daly S. The prevention of gestational diabetes mellitus with antenatal oral inositol supplementation: A randomized controlled trial. Diabetes Care. 2017;**40**(6):759-763

[29] He J, Zhang YL, Wang LP, Liu XC. Impact of different stereoisomers of inositol on insulin sensitivity of gestational diabetes mellitus patients. World Journal of Clinical Cases. 2021;**9**(3):565-572

[30] Di Biase M, Martinelli M, Florio V, Meldolesi C, Bonito M. The effectivnes of D-chiro inositol tretment in gestational diabetes. Diabetes Case Reports. 2017;**2**:3

Chapter 8

Exercise Interventions for the Management of Polycystic Ovary Syndrome (PCOS): An Update of the Literature

Lisa Vizza

Abstract

Polycystic Ovary Syndrome (PCOS) affects 6–10% women of reproductive age, and the diagnosis requires two of the three criteria: (1) menstrual irregularity; (2) polycystic ovaries on ultrasound; (3) elevated hormones (such as testosterone). Approximately 50–70% women have underlying insulin resistance and/or have a body mass index (BMI) greater than 28.0 kg/m^2, and if not managed, it can worsen the symptoms of PCOS. The first line of treatment for PCOS includes lifestyle management such as diet and/or exercise. Previous studies evaluated interventions such as aerobic, aerobic plus resistance and high intensity aerobic. These interventions formed part of the initial guidelines for the management of PCOS, although the guidelines did not include recommendations of resistance training in isolation. More recently, new studies have emerged which assessed resistance training interventions in isolation in PCOS, where these findings led to an update in the guidelines in PCOS to recommend resistance training as part of the management. The chapter will look to provide an update of the exercise literature in PCOS, as well as provide recommendations for future research.

Keywords: Polycystic Ovary Syndrome, lifestyle interventions, women's health, resistance exercise, aerobic exercise

1. Introduction

Polycystic Ovary Syndrome (PCOS) is a common endocrine condition, and affects approximately 6–10% of women during the reproductive years [1]. The diagnosis of PCOS requires two of the following three items as per the Rotterdam criteria: 1: menstrual irregularities (i.e., oligomenorrhea, amenorrhea); 2: polycystic ovaries on ultrasound; 3: androgen excess (i.e., elevated testosterone levels) [2].

The pathophysiology of PCOS is complex. Possible mechanisms include genetics, environmental and transgenerational factors, and can affect metabolic, reproductive and psychological outcomes [3, 4]. Insulin resistance may also be involved in the pathophysiology of PCOS [5, 6], where elevated levels may worsen features of PCOS (e.g., androgens, menstrual irregularity, and reproductive outcomes such as follicular arrest). A high proportion may also have underlying insulin resistance (50–70%) [7] and can be present in both overweight and non-overweight women with PCOS [5]. Interestingly, recent studies have also proposed a possible related intrinsic insulin resistance that are noted in PCOS versus their control counterparts [5].

Women with PCOS may also demonstrate an elevated body mass index (BMI) (>50% with BMI >25.0 kg/m^2) [8] infertility (70–80%) [9], and may also be at risk of future chronic diseases (e.g., cancer, cardiovascular disease, and diabetes) [10]. Anxiety and depression are also noted in this cohort (26–52%) [11], which can negatively affect quality of life [12, 13].

The first line treatment for the management of PCOS includes lifestyle modifications such as diet and/or exercise. Previous guidelines recommend 150 minutes of exercise per week, of which 90 minutes should be at a moderate to high intensity [14]. These guidelines were formed in accordance to previous literature which assessed aerobic, resistance and/or aerobic with a dietary component, and high intensity exercise. The initial guidelines did not include recommendations for resistance training as part of the management of PCOS. No studies were available at the time which evaluated this modality in isolation. The benefits of this intervention, such as improved insulin sensitivity and body composition which has been reported in previous diabetes studies [15, 16], could also be beneficial for the management of PCOS.

This limitation led to future studies to evaluate this intervention in isolation, which included both a feasibility study in women with PCOS [17], as well as other studies which incorporated various prescriptions, and these findings will be explored further in this chapter. The reported benefits led to a revision in the guidelines, to recommend resistance training as part of the management for PCOS [18].

The next sections will look to review the different types of intervention studies in PCOS, as well as provide directions for future research.

2. Exercise interventions in PCOS

2.1 Aerobic interventions-moderate and/or high intensity intermittent, and lifestyle interventions

Aerobic exercise is defined as an activity that uses large muscle groups, is maintained for a continuous time, and is rhythmic in nature [19]. Previous studies in PCOS assessed interventions such as cycle ergometry or treadmill for three to five sessions a week of 30–60 minutes at 60–70% of VO_{2max} and/or HR_{max} [20–29], self-selected or self-monitored (i.e. walking, cycle ergometry, treadmill) [30, 31], tailored intervention at an exercise dose of 14 kcal/kg/week) [32], walking and/or jogging [33–36], and interventions that were either moderate and/or high intensity exercise [37–49]. In addition, lifestyle and/or home-based interventions were also assessed in women with PCOS [50–61].

The interventions ranged from 4 to 52 weeks, and were compared to groups that received no training, diet, education, medication, lifestyle plus medication, or electroacupuncture. Sample size across studies ranged between 8 to 183 participants. Limited studies are available that incorporated a long-term follow-up component (>1 year). Outcomes ranged from anthropometric, cardiorespiratory, hematological, menstrual cyclicity, and hemodynamic. Further, recent studies also included other measurements such as quality of life (i.e., anxiety and depression using either the

Hospital Anxiety and Depression Scale (HADS), Polycystic Ovary Syndrome Questionnaire (PCOSQ), Short Form-36 (SF-36)) gene expression, enzymes, protein abundance, and a detailed list of all of these outcomes are reported in **Table 1**.

Adherence rates ranged between 60% and 100% across interventions that used cycling or ramp protocols, self-selected or self-monitored exercise (i.e., walking or a goal of 150 minutes of exercise a week), or a combination of moderate and/or high intensity aerobic exercise [24, 26, 27, 29, 32, 37, 40–42, 48, 50, 51, 73]. Further, adherence was also reported in other ways across studies which included weekly increase (e.g., 21.1%) [60], mean participation per week [58], and levels (e.g. high,

Moderate					
Author, Study design	**N enrolled (E) and completed (C)**	**Duration (weeks)**	**Intervention**	**Outcomes**	**Significant findings associated with exercise only**
Randeva et al. [34], Liao et al. [62] NRCT	E = 21 C = 12	24	Walking 20–60 min 3 sessions/wk. Volume increased fortnightly (120–420 min)	*Hemotological* FAI, folate, B12, homocysteine, creatinine, T_4, insulin, C, tg *Cardiorespiratory* VO_{2max} *Hemodynamic* SPB, DPB *Anthropometric* BMI, WHR *Other measurements* BDDE-SR	Homocysteine, WHR, VO_{2max}
Vigorito et al. RCT [29]	E = 90 C = 90	12	a. Cycle ergometer, 30 min at 60–70% of VO_{2max}, 3 sessions/wk. b. Control	*Hemotological* LH, FSH, PRL, E_2, P, 17-OHP, T, A, DHEA-S, SHBG, FAI, Hb, LDL, HDL, TC, fasting glucose, fasting insulin, AUC_{GLU}, AUC_{INS}, CRP *Cardiorespiratory* VO_{2max}, VO_{2AT}, VE/VCO_{2slope}, RER_{peak}, $Watt_{max}$ HRrest, HRpeak *Hemodynamic* SBPrest, SBPpeak, DBPrest, DBPpeak, HRR *Anthropometric* BMI, WHR, WC *Questionnaire* LTPA	BMI, WC, WHR, fasting insulin, AUC_{INS}, AUC_{GLU}/AUC_{INS}, VE/VCO_{2slope}, HRrest, SBPrest, DBPpeak, VO_{2max}, VO_{2AT}, peak workload, LTPA
Giallauria et al., NRCT [24]	E = 124 C = 124	12	a. Cycle ergometer, 30 min at 60–70% of VO_{2max}, 3 sessions/wk. b. Control	*Hemotological* LH, FSH, PRL, E_2, P, 17-OHP, T, A, DHEA-S, SHBG, FAI, Hb, LDL, HDL, TC, fasting glucose, fasting insulin, AUC_{GLU},	BMI, WHR, fasting insulin, AUC_{INS}, AUC_{INS}:AUC_{GLU}, CRP, WBC, VO_{2max}, VO_{2AT}, $Watt_{max}$, resting HR, post-exercise HHR

Moderate					
Author, Study design	**N enrolled (E) and completed (C)**	**Duration (weeks)**	**Intervention**	**Outcomes**	**Significant findings associated with exercise only**
				AUC_{INS}, AUC_{GLU}/ AUC_{INS}, CRP, WBC, neutrophils, lymphocytes *Cardiorespiratory* VO_{2max}, VO_{2AT}, VE/ VCO_{2slope}, RER_{peak}, $Watt_{max}$ HRrest, HRpeak *Hemodynamic* SBPrest, SBPpeak, DBPrest, DBPpeak, HRR *Anthropometric* BMI, WHR	
Palomba et al., NRCT [27]	E = 40 C = 40	24	a. Cycle ergometer, 30 min at 60–70% of VO_{2max}, 3 sessions/wk. b. Control	*Hemotological* LH, FSH, PRL, E_2, P, 17-OHP, T, A, DHEA-S, SHBG, FAI, TSH, fasting glucose, fasting insulin, GIR, HOMA-IR, $AUC_{glucose}$ *Menstrual cyclicity/ reproductive* Menses frequency, ovulation rate, ovulation frequency, pregnancy rate, abortion rate, cumulative ovulation rate, cumulative pregnancy rate *Anthropometric* BW, BMI, WC, WHR *Questionnaire* LTPA	LTPA (12 weeks), menses frequency, ovulation/ cumulative ovulation rate, abortion rate, trend higher pregnancy ($p = 0.075$), cumulative pregnancy ($p = 0.058$). BW, BMI, WC (12 weeks), T, SHBG, FAI (12 & 24 weeks) fasting insulin, GIR, HOMA-IR (12 & 24 weeks)
Brown et al., RCT [32]	E = 37 C = 20	24	8–12-week ramp +12 weeks exercise (14 kcal/kg/wk)	*Hemotological* T, fasting glucose, fasting insulin, 2 h glucose/insulin, HOMA-IR, AUC_{GLU}, AUC_{INS}, insulin sensitivity, HbA1c, VLDL/LDL/HDL particles, mean particle sizes (VLDL, LDL, HDL), lipids *Cardiorespiratory* VO_{2max} *Anthropometric*	VO_{2max}, trend AUCins ($p = 0.083$), tg ($p = 0.083$), large VLDL/chylomicrons ($p = 0.007$). Large HDL, medium/small HDL, HDL size, tg & VLDL tg, trend LDL particles ($p = 0.057$), HDL cholesterol ($p = 0.057$)

Moderate					
Author, Study design	**N enrolled (E) and completed (C)**	**Duration (weeks)**	**Intervention**	**Outcomes**	**Significant findings associated with exercise only**
				BW, BMI, WC, HC *Hemodynamic* SBP, DBP	
Stener-Victorin et al., RCT [36]	E = 23 C = 20	16	a. Low frequency electroacupuncture b. Walking 30–45 min 3 sessions/wk	*Hemotological* LH, FSH, total/free T, SHBG, FAI, DHEA-S, T_4, TSH, IGF-1, insulin, glucose, HOMA-IR, C, tg, HDL, LDL *Hemodynamic* SBP, DBP, HR *Anthropometric* BW, BMI, WHR, sagittal diameter *Sympathetic activity* MSNA *Menstrual cyclicity/ reproductive* Menstrual cycle status	MSNA burst activity and incidence, BMI, BW
Moro et al. [26] Covington et al. [22], Prospective study	E = 8 C = 8	16	Aerobic (treadmill), 5 sessions/wk. 55% VO_{2max}. Prescribed by exercise energy expenditure.	*Hemotological* Insulin sensitivity/ glucose disposal rate, FFA, fasting insulin, GDR, total T, FAI, SHBG, CRP, DHEA-S, WBC, HDL, LDL *Cardiorespiratory* $VO2_{max}$ *Anthropometric* BW, BMI, WHR, VF, FM, FFM, fat cell size, BF%, subcutaneous fat *Menstrual cyclicity/ reproductive* menstrual cyclicity (n follicles), ovarian morphology *Other measurements* Adipose tissue biopsy, β-adrenergic agonist, total RNA, isoproterenol (β-agonist) (A) and ANP (B), maximum postreceptor signaling agents, Dibutyryl-cAMP, Bromo-cGMP, MIF, IL-6, PAI-I, CD68, MCP-1, PLIN 1, 2, 3, 4, 5, ADP ribosylation factor	*Study also recruited 7 matched controls for baseline testing only* Insulin sensitivity (GDR), VO_{2max}, baseline lipolysis, lipolytic response to isoproterenol, lipolytic sensitivity, ANP maximal induced lipolysis, catecholamine lipolytic responsiveness, isoproterenol-induced lipid mobilization. FFA, total number follicles. PLIN3, ARF1, ARFRP1, BCOP and Sec23a

Moderate					
Author, Study design	**N enrolled (E) and completed (C)**	**Duration (weeks)**	**Intervention**	**Outcomes**	**Significant findings associated with exercise only**
				(e.g. ARF related protein 1), beta-coatomer, GDP exchange brefeldin A resistant factor 1, Sec23a, adipose triglyceride lipase, monoglyceride lipase, ATGL co activator	
Ladson et al., RCT [56]	E = 114 C = 38	24	a. Lifestyle and metformin b. Lifestyle and placebo Lifestyle = supervised (2× wk. was offered) and/or unsupervised (150 min aerobic exercise per wk)	*Hemotological* T, SHBG, FAI, E_2, LH, FSH, C, HDL, LDL, tg, fasting glucose, fasting insulin, AUC_{GLU}, AUC_{INS}, insulin sensitivity index, PDG *Cardiorespiratory* VO_{2max} *Hemodynamic* SBP, DBP *Anthropometric* BW, BMI, WC, BMD, total lean and fat, central abdominal fat, AbFM, central to total body ratio, BF% *Questionnaires* PCOSQ *Menstrual cyclicity/ reproductive* ovarian volume, follicle diameter, n ovulations	a. T, BW, insulin sensitivity b. SBP, AUC_{GLU}
Jedel et al. [30] Stener-Victorin et al. [36], RCT	E = 84 C = 72 *(Jedel=74)*	16 + 16wk f/up	a. Acupuncture b. Exercise (self-monitored, 30 min 3 sessions/wk) c. Control Exercise-brisk walking, cycling, other exercise	*Hemotological* T, FT, DHT, E1, E1-s, E_2, DHEA, DHEA-S, A, 5-DIOL, ADT-G, 3G, 17G, SHBG, LH, FSH *Cardiorespiratory* $VO2_{max}$ *Anthropometric* BMI, WHR *Questionnaire* MADRS-S, BSA-S, SF-36, PCOSQ *Menstrual cyclicity/ reproductive* Menstrual frequency	T, menstrual frequency, E1–2, 17G (wk 16). E_2 and 17G (week 32) SF-36 (role physical, physical functioning, general health) (wk 16). PCOSQ (emotion) (wk 16), (wk 32, infertility)

Moderate					
Author, Study design	**N enrolled (E) and completed (C)**	**Duration (weeks)**	**Intervention**	**Outcomes**	**Significant findings associated with exercise only**
Abazar et al., RCT [20]	E = 24 C = 24	12	a. Moderate, 3sessions/wk., 60–70% HR_{max} b. Control	*Hemotological* HDL, LDL, tg, VLDL, C *Anthropometric* BMI, WHR, BF%, BW	BMI, WHR, BF%, HDL, Tg
Sprung et al., Observational	E = 11 C = 6 *Study also recruited 6 matched control*	16	Moderate 3× wk. 30% HRR	*Hemotological* LH, FSH, P, E_2, T, FAI, SHBG, ALT, glucose, insulin, HOMA-IR, C, tg, HDL, LDL *Cardiorespiratory* $VO2_{max}$ *Anthropometric* BW, WC *Hemodynamic* SBP, DBP, HR *Other measurements* NO mediated microvascular function (local heating)	VO_{2max}, NO mediated microvascular function
De Frène et al., Prospective, longitudinal [52]	E = 31 C = 23	24	Exercise, diet (mild energy restriction), psychological subprogram Exercise = tailored to improve step count	*Anthropometric* BMI, BW, height *Questionnaire* PCOSQ, VAS	Total PCOSQ score, PCOSQ domains (emotions, body hair, weight, and infertility problems), VAS
Orio et al. [63] RCT	E = 150 C = 136	24	a. Oral contraceptive b. Exercise (3× wk. 45 min 60–70% VO_{2max}) c. Polyvitamin	*Hemotological* C, HDL, LDL, PAI-I, CRP, LH, FSH, TSH, PRL, E_2, P, 17-OHP, T, A, DHEA-S, SHBG, FAI, glucose, insulin, GIR, HOMA, $AUC_{glucose}$, $AUC_{insulin}$, $AUC_{glucose}$/ $AUC_{insulin}$ *Cardiorespiratory* $VO2_{max}$ *Anthropometric* BW, WHR *Hemodynamic* SBP, DBP *Menstrual cyclicity/ reproductive* Menstrual frequency *Other measurements* FMD, IMT	Exercise IMT, FMD, HDL, CRP, PAI-I, VO_{2max}, BMI, WHR, HOMA-IR, AUC_{ins}, menstrual frequency
Al-Eisa et al., NRCT [21]	E = 90 C = 90	12	Treadmill walking, 45 min, 3 sessions/wk. 65–75%	*Hemotological* FSH, E_2, PRL, AMH, adiponectin, fasting glucose, fasting	*Study included:* *GA-Control BMI 20–29* *GB- PCOS BMI 30–*

Moderate					
Author, Study design	**N enrolled (E) and completed (C)**	**Duration (weeks)**	**Intervention**	**Outcomes**	**Significant findings associated with exercise only**
				insulin, GIR, HOMA-IR, AFC *Cardiorespiratory* $VO2_{max}$ *Hemodynamic* SBP, DBP *Anthropometric* BMI, BW, WHR, WC *Menstrual cyclicity/ reproductive* Ovulation rate, menstrual cyclicity	*35* *GC- Obese BMI 30–35* **GB and GC** BMI, BW, WC, WHR, PRL, fasting glucose/insulin, HOMA-IR, FSH, E_2, GIR, adiponectin, AMH, AFC, ovulation rate, menstrual cyclicity
Gilani et al. [64] RCT	E = 40 C = 40	8	a. Running 3× wk. 60–75% $HR_{max.}$ b. Control	*Hemotological* PRL, LH, FSH, DHEA-S, AMH, A, 17-OHP, T, P, E_2, FAI *Anthropometric* BMI, WHR	LH, PRL, A
McBreairty et al. [65] RCT	E = 95 C = 61	16	All px underwent TLC diet for 2 weeks a. Exercise and pulse base diet b. Exercise and TLC diet Exercise-aerobic 5× wk., 3 sessions supervised, self-selected 60% HR_{max}	*Hemotological* E_2, T *Anthropometric* BMI, BW, FM, LM, BF%, BMC	BMI, BW, FM, BMD
Kazemi et al. [66] RCT	E = 95 C = 25	16 + 6–12-month f/ up	a. Exercise and pulse base diet b. Exercise and TLC diet Exercise-aerobic 5× wk. 45 min 60–75% HR_{max}	*Hemotological* T, SHBG, FAI, LH, FSH, FAI *Menstrual cyclicity/ reproductive* Ovarian morphology, menstrual cycle length	Ovarian morphology, FAI, menstrual cyclicity
Wu et al. 2021 [67] RCT	E = 38 C = 38	12	a. Aerobic 4× wk. 30 min b. Control	*Hemotological* Glucose, C, HDL, LDL, tg, Cr, FSH, LH, T, DHEA-S, AMH, MDA *Cardiorespiratory* $VO2_{max}$ *Hemodynamic* SBP, DBP *Anthropometric* BMI, BW *Other measurements* Oxidative stress	BMI, VO_{2max}, AMH, oxidative stress

Moderate					
Author, Study design	**N enrolled (E) and completed (C)**	**Duration (weeks)**	**Intervention**	**Outcomes**	**Significant findings associated with exercise only**
Upasana et al., RCT [61]	E = 60 C = 48	20	a. Home based aerobic training b. Control Home based- 5×/wk. 30 min (brisk walking, cycling)	*Hemotological* Fasting glucose, fasting insulin, HOMA-IR, CRP *Anthropometric* BW, BMI, WC, HC	BW, BMI, WC, HC, fasting glucose, CRP, HOMA-IR
Ramanjaneya et al., NRCT, [28]	E = 21 C = 21	8	Treadmill exercise 3 sessions/wk for 1 hr, 60% VO_{2max}	*Hemotological* PG, insulin, NEFA, T, FAI, SHBG, LH, FSH, C, Tg, HDL, LDL, ALT, HbA1c, TSH, DHEA-S, A *Cardiorespiratory* $VO2_{max}$ *Hemodynamic* SBP, DBP *Anthropometric* BW, BMI, WC, HC *Other measurements* Complement related proteins (C1q, C3, C3b/lC3b, C4, Factor-B and H, properdin, C2, C4b, C5, C5a, D, mannose binding lectin, factor 1)	*Study recruited PCOS and matched controls.* N.S

Moderate and/or high intensity					
Author, Study design	**N enrolled (E) and completed (C)**	**Duration (weeks)**	**Intervention**	**Outcomes**	**Significant findings associated with exercise only**
Hutchinson et al., 2011, 2012 Harrison et al., 2012., Moran et al., 2011, prospective exercise intervention	E = 34 C = 21	12	3 sessions/wk 1 hr. Alternated between 1. 60 min moderate-intensity treadmill walking/jogging 75–85% HR_{max} 2. High intensity and intermittent exercise (6 × 5 min with 2-min recovery 95–100% HR_{max})	*Hemotological* T, SHBH, FAI, fasting glucose, fasting insulin, GIR, HOMA, HbA1c, C, TC, HDL, LDL, triglycerol, FAI, IFG, tg *Cardiorespiratory* $VO2_{max}$, RER, HR_{max} *Hemodynamic* SBP, DBP *Anthropometric* lean tissue mass, FM, AbFM, VF, SCFAT, BF%, BW, BMI, WC, WHR, thigh muscle attenuation. *Protein abundance*	*Trial recruited both PCOS and matched controls* *PCOS* BMI, VF, IR, Tg, trend lower PGC1A and higher PGC1A protein abundance, BW, WC, GIR, trend for CT muscle attenuation, $VO2_{max}$, total and AbFM, AMH *Non PCOS* WC, SCFAT, $VO2_{max}$

Moderate and/or high intensity					
Author, Study design	**N enrolled (E) and completed (C)**	**Duration (weeks)**	**Intervention**	**Outcomes**	**Significant findings associated with exercise only**
				PGC1α, complex I, II, III, IV, V *Enzyme* ß-HAD, CS *Gene expression* PGC1A, TFAM, NRF1, COX4	
Kostrzewa-Nowak et al., 2014, NRCT [25]	E = 34 C = 34	12	1. Familiarization (3 sessions/wk. 30 min, 50% HR_{max}) 2. Exercise = 60 min low-high impact 4 phases % HR_{max} (3 weeks each): 50–60%, 55–65%, 60–70%, 65–75%	*Hemotological* WBC, RBC, Hb, HTC, MCV, MCH, MCHC, PLT tg, C, HDL, LDL *Cardiorespiratory* VO_{2max}, V_{E2max}, HR_{max}, VO_2/AT *Anthropometric* Skinfolds- thoracical, abdomen, subscapularis, triceps, and crus BW, BMI, FFM, BF %, TBW, BMR	Results reported by BMI: *Underweight*: BMI and weight, VO_{2max} *Normal weight*: n.s *Overweight*: BMI, skinfolds, weight, TBW, BF%, Tg, C, HDL, LDL, V_{Emax}
Gaeini et al., 2014, RCT [39]	E = 40 C = 40	12	a. 3 session/wk. 25–30 min, 60–85% HR_{max} b. Control	*Hemotological* 17-OHP, DHEA-S *Anthropometric* BW *Menstrual cyclicity/ reproductive* Menstrual cycle status, follicles	*Recruited lean and obese PCOS.* *Obese PCOS* DHEA-S,17-OHP, BW *Both groups* Follicles, menstrual cycle status
Sa et al., 2016, RCT [35]	E = 30 C = 30	16	a. Walking/ jogging 3 sessions/wk. 40 min b. Usual care 4 phases % HR_{max} (monthly increments) 60–70%, 70–75%, 75–80%, 80–85%	*Hemotological* FSH, LH, T, DHEA-S, insulin *Cardiorespiratory* VO_{2max} *Hemodynamic* HRV, BP, HR, HR_{max} *Anthropometric* BMI	HR, SBP, HRV
Costa et al., 2017, two-way parallel controlled trial [33]	E = 30 C = 27	16	a. 3 sessions/ wk = 40 min walking and/ or jogging (outdoor track). intensity HR_{max} b. Control	*Hemotological* DHEA-S, LH, FSH, TC, HDL, LDL, TG, FG, 2-H-PG, AUC OGTT, insulin, log insulin, HOMA-IR, IL-6, TN-F, CRP *Anthropometric* BMI, WC *Cardiorespiratory* VO_{2peak}, HR_{max} *Hemodynamic*	SF-36 (physical functioning, general health, mental health), VO_{2peak}, BMI, WC, SBP, DBP, mean BP, total cholesterol, LDL, TNF-alpha, CRP. Mean HR 4 different phases.

Moderate and/or high intensity					
Author, Study design	**N enrolled (E) and completed (C)**	**Duration (weeks)**	**Intervention**	**Outcomes**	**Significant findings associated with exercise only**
				SBP, DBP *Questionnaires* SF-36	
Scott et al., 2017, NRCT [49]	E = 16 C = 16	12	3 sessions/ wk 1 hr. Alternating: 1. 20–60 min walking/jogging, 75–80% HR_{max} with 2-min recovery 2. HITT (6–8, 5 min intervals, 95–100% HR_{max} with 2-min recovery) Wk 4 = 8 intervals, 1 min rest	*Hemotological* Glucose, log insulin, HOMA-IR, GIR/FFM *Cardiorespiratory* VO_{2max} *Anthropometric* BMI, FFM, FM, android/gynoid fat, android/gynoid ratio	*Study recruited PCOS and non PCOS* VO_{2max}, trend towards decrease BF %
Kogure et al., 2020, [43], Lopes et al., 2018 [44] RCT	E = 110 C = 89	16	a. CAT- 3 sessions/wk. 30 min 65–80% HR_{max} b. IAT-3 sessions/wk., 30 min (2 min high intensity 70–90% HR_{max} separated by 3 min recovery (60–70%)) c. Control	*Hemotological* T, FAI, SHBG *Anthropometric* Height, BW, WC, HC, WHR, BMI *Questionnaire* HADS, FRS, FSRI, dis (satisfaction grade)	Dis (satisfaction) grade, total FSFI, HADS.
Ribeiro et al., 2019, [47] RCT	E = 110 C = 87	16	a. CAT-3 sessions/wk. 30 min 65–80% HR_{max} b. IAT-3 sessions/ wk. 30 min (2 min high intensity 70–90% HR_{max} separated by 3 min recovery (60–70%) c. Control	*Hemotological* T, PRL, TSH, 17 OHP *Anthropometric* BMI, WC, WHR *Menstrual cyclicity/ reproductive* Ovarian morphology *Questionnaire* SF-36	*CAT* WC, HC, WHR, SF-36 (physical functioning, role physical, general health, social role, emotional role, mental health) *IAT* WHR, SF-36 (physical functioning, role physical, general health, vitality, social role, emotional role, mental health) *IAT and CAT* T
Faryadian et al., 2019, [38] Quasi experimental design	E = 24 C = 24	12	a. HITT-3 sessions/wk. 2 sessions- 4 × 4 min 90–95% HR_{max} and 3×	*Hemotological* Fasting glucose, fasting insulin, HOMA-IR, CRP *Anthropometric* BW, BMI	CRP, HOMA-IR

Moderate and/or high intensity					
Author, Study design	**N enrolled (E) and completed (C)**	**Duration (weeks)**	**Intervention**	**Outcomes**	**Significant findings associated with exercise only**
			moderate intensity running, 70% HR_{max}, 1 session- 10×1 min high intensity running, 10×1 min rest. b. Control		
Benham et al., 2020 [37], RCT	E = 47 C = 40	24 (+ 24 wk. f/up)	a. HITT 3 sessions/wk., 10×30s 90% HRR or 9/10 Borg, alternate with 90s low intensity b. CAT (3 sessions/wk., 40 min moderate 50–60% HRR or 6/10 Borg) c. Control	*Hemotological* HbA1c, fasting insulin, fasting glucose, HOMA-IR, C, LDL, HDL, Tg, ALT, GGT *Cardiorespiratory* VO_{2max} *Anthropometric* BMI, weight, WC *Hemodynamic* SBP, DBP	BMI (CAT), WC (control and HITT), fasting glucose (HITT), LDL (HITT), HDL (HITT)
Elbandrawy et al., 2022, RCT [23]	E = 40 C = 40	12	a. 3 sessions/wk., 30 min treadmill (10 min low intensity, 20 min moderate (60–70% HR_{max})) + Metformin (1500 mg) b. Metformin (1500 mg)	*Hemotological* IL-6, TNFα, CRP *Anthropometric* BMI	IL-6, TNFα, CRP
Philbois et al., 2022, [68] RCT	E = 110 C = 75	16	a. CAT-3×wk 60 min, 70–80% HRR b. HITT-2 min 85–90% HRR, and 3 min 65–70% HRR c. Control	*Hemotological* Insulin, glucose, tg, C, HOMA-IR, HDL, LDL *Cardiorespiratory* VO_{2max} *Anthropometric* BMI, weight *Hemodynamic* SBP, DBP, HR, HRV	HR, VO_{2max}, T
Mohammadi et al., 2023 [45] RCT	E = 30 C = 28	8	a. HITT-3 sessions/wk. low intensity run (50% max	*Hemotological* Fasting glucose, insulin, HOMA-IR, QUICKI, LDL, HDL, total C, tg, A/P, TS/C	BMI, WHR, visceral fat, insulin, insulin resistance, LDL, atherogenic index, cholesterol, cortisol

Moderate and/or high intensity					
Author, Study design	**N enrolled (E) and completed (C)**	**Duration (weeks)**	**Intervention**	**Outcomes**	**Significant findings associated with exercise only**
			speed) and 3×30s sprint followed by 30s slow running. b. Control 3rd week = 6 sets	ratio *Cardiorespiratory* VO_{2max} *Anthropometric* BW, BMI, BF%, WHR, VAT, VAI	
Samadi et al., 2023 [69], RCT	E = 30 C = 30	12	a. HITT- 3× wk. 30 min (4×4 min, 8 rounds 20s all out and 10s rest (80–85% HR_{max}) and Metformin (1500 mg) b. Metformin (1500 mg)	*Hemotological* HOMA-IR, SHBG, T, LH, DHEA-S, FSH, FAI *Cardiorespiratory* VO_{2max} *Anthropometric* FM, BMI, WHR, HC *Menstrual cyclicity/ reproductive* Ovarian morphology, menstrual cyclicity	BMI, FM FSH, T, SHBG, HOMA-IR
Lifestyle interventions					
Author, Study design	N enrolled (E) & analyzed (A)	Duration (weeks)	Intervention	Outcomes	Significant findings associated with exercise only
Guzick et al., 1994, [70] RCT	E = 12 C = 12	12	a. Behavior weight control b. Control Guidance provided to improve physical activity levels	*Hemotological* T, SHBG, fasting insulin, glucose, LH *Anthropometric* BW	BW, SHBG, trend fasting insulin
Hoeger et al., 2004, [54] RCT	E = 38 C = 23	48	a. Metformin (1700 mg) b. Lifestyle and placebo c. Lifestyle and Metformin d. Placebo Lifestyle: nutrition (500–1000 deficit), behavior, exercise (150 min per wk)	*Hemotological* SHBG, insulin, glucose, T, FAI, AUC_{GLU}, AUC_{INS}, fasting insulin *Anthropometric* BW, BMI, WHR, WC *Other measurements* Weekly urine samples (pregnanediol)	BW, T, FAI, trend fasting glucose
Pasquali et al. 2011 [71], NRCT	E = 100 C = 65	24	Diet (hypocaloric 1200–1200 kcal day) followed by mildly restricted intake (500 kcal day deficit), walking 30 min 5× wk	*Hemotological* T, SHBG, FAI, A, DHEA-S, 17-OHP, LH, FSH, LH/FSH, E_2, LDL, HDL, tg, fasting glucose, fasting insulin, HOMA-IR, QUICKI, C, $ISI_{composite}$	WC, A, 17-OHP, LH, C, HDL, tg, fasting glucose, fasting insulin, HOMA-IR, QUICKI, $ISI_{composite}$

Moderate and/or high intensity					
Author, Study design	**N enrolled (E) and completed (C)**	**Duration (weeks)**	**Intervention**	**Outcomes**	**Significant findings associated with exercise only**
				Anthropometric BMI, WC, HC, WHR *Menstrual cyclicity/ reproductive* Menses, ovarian morphology/volume, follicle number	
Mahoney et al. 2013 [58], Prospective quantitative design	E = 12 C = 9	12	a. Lifestyle (3–5 sessions/wk., 30–60 min, low impact exercises (walking, cycling), RX 2 to 3 sessions. b. Counseling- every 2 weeks (6 sessions total)	*Anthropometric* BMI *Menstrual cyclicity/ reproductive* Menstrual history *Questionnaire* Block Brief food frequency, Block physical activity screener. *Other measurements* Diet modification (energy intake, fat, saturated fat, carbohydrates, protein)	Weight, mean daily calorie, fat and carbohydrate intake, frequency home or gym exercise, menstrual cyclicity 50% among prior amenorrheic patients.
Konopka et al., 2015 [55], RCT	E = 39 C = 39	12	a. Lean PCOS-control b. Obese PCOS-Aerobic c. Obese PCOS-control Exercise = Supervised: 60 min HR 65% VO_{2peak} 5× wk.	*Hemotological* Glucose, insulin, HOMA, c-peptide, P, E_2 *Cardiorespiratory* VO_{2peak} *Anthropometric* BMI, BW, FM, FFM *Other measurements* Hyperinsulinemic-euglycaemic pancreatic clamp (insulin sensitivity), muscle biopsy (vastus lateralis), mitochondrial respiration (complex I, complex I and II, complex II, FCCP, O2flux (state 3 (CI), cytoc, State 3 (CI + II), state 3 (CII), state 4, FCCP, antimycin A), respiratory control ratio (RCR), phosphorylation efficiency (ADP:O), H_2O_2). H_2O_2 production,	*Study recruited obese and lean PCOS* State 4, ADP:O, mtH2O2 emissions, VO_{2peak}, maximal citrate synthase activity, maximal mitochondrial oxidative activity, RCR and ADP:O, H2O2-emitting potential of isolated mitochondria, mtH2O2, catalyze activity, GIR, insulin sensitivity, AUC_{GLU}

Moderate and/or high intensity					
Author, Study design	**N enrolled (E) and completed (C)**	**Duration (weeks)**	**Intervention**	**Outcomes**	**Significant findings associated with exercise only**
				antioxidant activity and mRNA expression (catalyze activity, SOD), oxidative damage (8-oxo-dG), mtDNA	
Legro et al., 2015, [57] Dokras et al., 2016 [53], RCT	E = 149 C = 132	16	a. OCP b. Lifestyle (caloric restriction, weight loss medication, exercise) c. OCP + lifestyle	*Hemotological* AMH, T, SHBG, C, HDL, LDL, Tg, OGTT, AUC insulin, AUC glucose, insulin, *Anthropometric* BW, BMI, WC, FM, lean mass, BF% *Hemodynamic* SBP, DBP *Questionnaire* PCOSQ, 3-day diet log, SF-36	BW, cumulative ovulation rates, SF-36 (general health all groups), lifestyle only (vitality), PCOSQ (OCP and combined improvement in all domains, LS- not in hair and emotional)
Nagelberg et al., 2016 [60], RCT	E = 21 C = 21	4	a. Pedometer b. Control Step goal- increase 50% per wk. All received clomiphene	*Hemotological* HbA1c, fasting glucose, TSH, Vit D, T, DHEA-S *Anthropometric* BMI	N.S due to small sample size. 7 became pregnant (4 in intervention and 3 in control), 50% intervention group lost weight and only 3/10 patients achieved step count.
Arentz et al., 2017 [50], RCT	E = 122 C = 102	12	a. Lifestyle b. Lifestyle and herbal medicine Lifestyle = 150 min wk.	*Hemotological* FSH, LH, E_2, T, SHBG, FAI, fasting glucose, fasting insulin *Anthropometric* BMI, WC, WHR *Hemodynamic* SBP, DBP *Questionnaires* PCOSQ, DASS-21 *Menstrual cyclicity/ reproductive* Oligomenorrhea	Oligomenorrhea, BMI, insulin, LH, BP, PCOSQ, DASS-21, pregnancy rates (Lifestyle and herbal medicine)
Cooney et al., 2018 [51], RCT	E = 33 C = 24	16	a. CBT b. No CBT All received 30 min weekly nutrition/ exercise counseling. Exercise goal = 50 min and increase to 175 min per wk	*Hemotological* C, HDL, LDL, tg, fasting glucose, insulin, HOMA-IR, total/free T, SHBG, CRP, IL6, apolipoprotein A1 and B *Anthropometric* BW, BMI, WC, HC,	BW, PCOSQ (more in CBT). STAI and CES-D, Total/free T. Heart rate response (greater in CBT)

Moderate and/or high intensity					
Author, Study design	**N enrolled (E) and completed (C)**	**Duration (weeks)**	**Intervention**	**Outcomes**	**Significant findings associated with exercise only**
				WHR *Hemodynamic* SBP, DBP, heart rate response *Questionnaires* CES-D, STAI, PSS, ACE, PCOSQ, TSST	
Manteghi et al., 2021 [59], RCT	E = 120 C = 104	24	a. Letrozole 2× evening, HMG injection, aerobic exercise 3× wk 30 min b. Two letrozole tablets	*Hemotological* FBS, HbA1c, FSH, LH, E_2, PRL, TSH *Anthropometric* BMI *Menstrual cyclicity/ reproductive* Number follicles, pregnancy rates, rate live births	Pregnancy rates, rate live births, HbA1c and fasting blood sugar
De loos et al. 2023, [72] RCT	E = 183 C = 76	52	a. Lifestyle with sms support b. Lifestyle c. Usual care Lifestyle = encouraged to exercise 5× wk. 30 min, and 8–10 rx exercises 2x wk	*Cardiorespiratory* VO_{2max}, peak workload *Anthropometric* BMI, BW *Questionnaire* IPAQ	Lifestyle and sms-IPAQ, peak workload

Abbreviations: T, testosterone; SHBG, sex hormone binding globulin; E_2, estradiol; LH, luteinizing hormone; FSH, follicle stimulating hormone; P, progesterone; DHEA-S, dehydroepiandrosterone; A, Androstenedione; 17-OHP, 17-Hydroxyprogesterone; FAI, free androgen index; PRL, prolactin; TSH, thyroid stimulating hormone; PDG, pregnanediol-3-glucoronide; C, cholesterol; TC, total cholesterol; Tg, triglycerides; LDL, low density lipoprotein; HDL, high density lipoprotein; VLDL, very low density lipoprotein; Hb, hemoglobin; HOMA-IR, homeostatic model assessment insulin resistance; QUICKI, quantitative insulin-sensitivity check index; GIR, glucose infusion rate; $AUC_{GLU/INS}$, Area under curve glucose/insulin; IGF-1, insulin growth factor; T_4, thyroxine; CRP, C-reactive protein; WBC, white blood cells; NMR, nuclear magnetic resonance spectroscopy; BMI, body mass index; BF%, body fat percentage; FM, fat mass; FFM, fat free mass; AbFm, abdominal fat mass; SCFAT, subcutaneous fat; WC, waist circumference; WHR, waist to hip ratio; HC, hip circumference; SO2S, sum of 2 skinfolds; REE, resting energy expenditure; SBP, systolic blood pressure; DBP, diastolic blood pressure; LTPA, leisure time physical activity; HbA1c, glycated hemoglobin; HR, heart rate; HRR, heart rate reserve; VO_{2max}, maximal oxygen consumption; VO_{2AT}, maximal oxygen consumption at anaerobic threshold; VE/VCO_{2slope}, minute ventilation-carbon dioxide production; AER+RX, aerobic plus resistance; RCT, randomized control trial; RM, repetition maximum; NRCT, non randomized control trial; BDDE-SR, body dysmorphic disorder examination; BW, body weight; FFA, free fatty acid; BMD, bone mineral density; PCOSQ, Polycystic Ovary Syndrome Questionnaire; E1, estrone; E1-s, E1 sulphate; 5-DIOL, 5-androstene-3; ADT-G, androsterone glucuronide; 3G, androstane-3; 17G, 17-diol-17 glucuronide; MADRS-S, Montgomery Åsberg Depression Rating Scale; BSA-S, Brief Scale for Anxiety; SF-36, Short form-36; AFC, Antral follicle count; NS, not significant; NEFA, non esterified free fatty acids; RBC, red blood cell; HTC, hematocrit; MCV, mean corpuscular volume; MCH, mean corpuscular hemoglobin; MCHC, mean corpuscular hemoglobin concentration; PTL, platelets total level; TBW, total body water; BMR, basal metabolic rate; HRV, heart rate variability; CAT, continuous aerobic training; IAT, intermittent aerobic training; FSRI, Female sexual function index; FRS, figure rating scale; HITT, high intensity interval training; GGT, gamma-glutamyl transferase; ALT, alanine aminotransferase; A/P, Atherogenic index of plasma; TS/C, testosterone to cortisol ratio; VAT, visceral adipose tissue; VAI, visceral adiposity index; CES-D, Center for Epidemiologic Studies Depression Scale; STAI, State-Trait Anxiety Inventory; PSS, perceived stress scale; ACE, adverse childhood experience; TSST, Trier Social stress test; DASS-21, depression anxiety and stress score; IFG, impaired fasting glucose; RER, respiratory exchange ratio; PLT, platelets total level; GDR, glucose disposal rate; IL-6, interleukin-6; MIF, Covinton-Macrophage inhibitory factor; PAI-I, plasminogen activator inhibitor; CD68, cluster of differentiation marker 68; MCP-1, monocyte chemotactic protein-1; IPAQ, international physical activity questionnaire; MSNA, muscle sympathetic nerve activity; AMH, anti-Mullarian hormone; MDA, malondialdehyde; HADS, hospital anxiety and depression scale; TNFα, tumor necrosis factor; PLIN, Perilipin.

Table 1.
Summary exercise studies (aerobic, moderate and/or high intensity, lifestyle interventions).

moderate and low) [27], or there were a few studies that did not report this [20, 21, 23, 25, 28, 33–36, 38, 39, 43–45, 47, 52, 54–57, 59, 61, 71].

Adverse event reporting was also not always reported across interventions [20–23, 25, 26, 32, 35, 36, 39, 49, 52, 73], and similarly, this was also the same for dropout rates [20, 21, 23–26, 29, 35, 39, 55, 73]. Of the studies that reported dropout rates, this ranged between 10% and 70% across interventions [5, 27, 30, 32, 34, 41–43, 47, 49–52, 54, 56, 59, 61], where higher dropout rates were reported for interventions that used metformin (>40% [54, 56]), walking (where the volume increased fortnightly-57% [34]), moderate to high intensity exercise (30–60%) [41, 42, 49], and 30 min weekly nutrition/exercise counseling (where one group also received cognitive behavioral therapy (54%)) [51]. Across studies, co interventions was not always reported. While limited studies are available that reported for differences in dropout rates between ethnic groups, interestingly, two studies reported a higher percentage/number in ethnic groups that dropped out from interventions such as lifestyle and metformin (76% versus 62%) [56], and a ramp plus 12-week exercise protocol (25%) [32].

Characteristics of participants recruited in these studies ranged between 20 to 35 years of age, and BMI > 25.0 kg/m^2. Most studies excluded participants with a history of the following which included but was not limited to, cardiovascular, metabolic, or glucose intolerance. Across studies, the main baseline characteristics that were reported included body composition, hematological, cardiovascular, but not all studies reported menstrual cycle status as a baseline characteristic in PCOS. Further items that were not reported (although it is possible some studies could have reported these separately as supplementary materials) included family history, PCOS phenotype, previous pregnancies, or other co morbid conditions such as metabolic syndrome. Further, limited studies have not included other baseline characteristics for example pain perception, where higher prevalence of pain perception has been reported in PCOS in a study using the SF-36, and may be associated with infertility, obesity, inflammation or insulin resistance) [74], as well as sleep disorders (this was reported in one study which included numbers of obstructive sleep apnea) which may be prevalent in this cohort [37, 75].

To our knowledge, only few studies recruited PCOS women with a BMI < 25.0 kg/m^2 [25, 39], and also, for studies that did not report this, it is unclear as to whether participants in various ethnic groups were recruited. For example, differences in PCOS symptoms (e.g., hyperandrogenism and metabolic symptoms) were noted between Hispanics versus non-Hispanics [76]. Of the two studies that reported higher dropout rates in this group, it would be important to determine as to whether additional strategies are required to improve compliance rates in this group. Further, not all studies reported other ethnicity outcomes such as English language proficiency and Ancestry. Furthermore, it is probable that participants with limited English proficiency requiring translation were also not included in these studies. A previous review reported that approximately 21% of studies excluded participants with low English proficiency from research [77]. Exclusion of these participants from research would not provide a true representation of the study population, particularly in countries such as Australia where the population is culturally diverse.

Overall, the benefits of aerobic interventions that used either moderate and/or a combination of moderate and high intensity in women with PCOS with a BMI > 28.0 kg/m^2 ranged from improved body composition (e.g., reduced waist circumference, waist to hip ratio and body weight), hematological (e.g., improved lipids, hormones, insulin sensitivity), cardiorespiratory and hemodynamic (e.g. aerobic fitness, blood pressure), menstrual cyclicity, and other outcomes (e.g., mRNA, protein abundance). Further, for recent studies, quality of life was also improved following an aerobic intervention, which included improved anxiety and depression scores (using HADS), PCOSQ (domains such as emotions, body hair, weight, and infertility problems), and quality of life (SF-36 on domains such as role physical, physical functioning, general health, and social role).

While further studies are warranted to investigate the benefits of aerobic exercise interventions in lean women with PCOS (BMI <28.0 kg/m^2), possible benefits may include a change in left/right follicles and menstrual cyclicity following moderate to high intensity exercise (60–85%) [39], as well as changes in BMI, weight and $VO2_{max}$ following low-high impact exercises at 50–75% HR_{max} [25].

A detailed list of outcomes for each of these studies and their findings are provided in **Table 1**.

2.2 Resistance interventions (with or without aerobic intervention)

Resistance training is a form of exercise that challenges the muscles with unaccustomed loads using free weights and/or machine weights. Resistance training has also been reviewed in studies in PCOS, either in isolation and/or combined with other modalities (e.g., aerobic, dietary component), and the studies incorporated exercises using free weights, machines, aqua aerobics, or Thera bands.

For studies that assessed aerobic and resistance, either in isolation or in combination, the exercise prescription was described across most interventions. For the aerobic intervention, this included 30 minutes on the treadmill/bike at 70–85% HR_{max} [78], 25–45 minutes at 60–80% HR_{max} [79], high intensity interval training (e.g. 4×30 s or 4×4 minutes at 90–100% maximum speed) [80–82], step routine (5–20 minutes) [83], goal oriented (200–300 minutes total per week) [84], or individually tailored [85]. For the resistance training, the prescription ranged from two to three sessions per week, with some studies prescribing a whole body intervention [81–83], while a number of studies did not describe the intervention in detail [78, 80, 84, 85]. The intensity of the resistance training interventions was determined by either repetitions (8–16 repetitions [78], % 1 Repetition Maximum (RM)) [79–82], Borg scale [83], or was not reported [78, 84–86].

Of the studies that assessed resistance training intervention only, two studies did not describe the intervention in detail [87, 88]. The prescription also varied across studies. For example, a study integrated macrocycles (e.g. four macrocycles (3 weeks of increased intensity, fourth week at a reduced intensity, and progressively increasing the intensity while reducing repetitions between sets (e.g. week 1–60%, 65%, 70%, 65%, week 2–65%, 70%, 75%, and 70%)) [89, 90], while another study used mesocycles (first 3 weeks performed for three sessions a week with the intensity increasing at 5% per week, and for the fourth week, sessions were performed for two sessions a week while the intensity reduced by 5% [47]. For another study, the intervention consisted of two supervised sessions per week of a whole-body routine with each exercise performed for three sets of 8–12 repetitions, and the weight was increased once the participant was able to perform three sets of the exercise at 8–12 repetitions, and it also included two supervised sessions at home using calisthenica [17].

The interventions ranged between 8 to 24 weeks, and most studies included comparator groups such as dietary restriction, no treatment (control), medication (e.g., metformin, calcium, clomiphene). Sample size across studies ranged between 8 to 143 participants. To the best of our knowledge, limited studies are available that included a long-term follow-up, and similar to the aerobic training studies, co interventions were not always reported. Outcomes ranged from anthropometric, cardiorespiratory, hematological, menstrual cyclicity, and hemodynamic. Further, these studies collected other measurements such as endothelial vasodilation, step count, quality of life (i.e., anxiety and depression), heart rate recovery and telomere content. The listed outcomes are provided in **Table 2**.

For the resistance training interventions, adherence rates were not always reported across all studies. Of those that reported this, this ranged between 70% to 90% for

Mixed interventions (aerobic and/or resistance)

Author, Study design	N enrolled (E) & completed (C)	Duration (weeks)	Intervention	Outcomes	Significant findings associated with exercise only
Bruner et al., 2006, [78] RCT	E = 12 C = 12	12	a. Nutrition counseling and AER + RX - 3× wk. 90 min (30 min TM or bike at 70–85% HR_{max}) and RX (12 exercises 3×15) b. Nutrition counseling	*Hemotological* T, SHBG, FAI, LH: FSH, fasting insulin, QUICKI *Cardiorespiratory* VO_{2max}, REE *Anthropometric* BW, BMI, WG, SO2S *Menstrual cyclicity/ reproductive* Ovarian follicle (left and right)	WG, SO2S, fasting insulin, VO_{2max}
Thomson et al., 2008, 2016, [79, 91] RCT	E = 94 C = 52	20	a. Diet + AER: walking/jogging 5 x wk. Wk 1 (25–30 min at 60–65% HR_{max}), and 45 min at 75–80% HR_{max} b. Diet + AER and RX same aerobic 3× wk., RX 2× wk. non consecutive. 5 exercises wks 1–2: 50–60% 1RM and increased to 65–75% 1RM. c. Diet only	*Hemotological* T, SHBG, FAI, C, LDL, HDL, tg, insulin, glucose, HOMA, urinary (PDG) *Cardiorespiratory* VO_{2peak} *Hemodynamic* SBP, DBP *Anthropometric* BF%, FM, FFM, AbFm WC *Menstrual cyclicity/ reproductive* Menstrual cyclicity *Questionnaires* PCOSQ, CES-D, EBBS	BP, fasting glucose, fasting insulin, HOMA, lipids, t, FAI, SHBG, ovulation, menstrual cyclicity (all groups), BF%, FM and FFM (exercise groups), trend AbFM ($p = 0.08$), EBBS, VO_{2peak}
Aubuchon et al., 2009, [84] open longitudinal study	E = 37 C = 33	14	Group exercise (AER + RX)-60 min. Group nutrition classes (90 min/ wk. for 4 weeks) 60 min session, Goal = 200–300 min/wk	*Anthropometric* BMI, WC, HC, BF% *Menstrual cyclicity/ reproductive* Clinical pregnancy rates	BF%, weight loss, BMI, WC, HC
Nybacka et al., 2011, [85] RCT	E = 57 C = 25	16	a. Diet b. Exercise c. Diet and exercise Diet: restriction ≥600 kcal/d Exercise: tailored	*Hemotological* FSH, LH, T, SHBG, fT, DHEA-S, 17-OHP, E_2, IGF-I, IGFBP-I, insulin, glucose, HOMA	Caloric intake/ 24 hrs, steps/d, weight, BF%, total lean body mass, T/SHBG ratio

Mixed interventions (aerobic and/or resistance)					
Author, Study design	**N enrolled (E) & completed (C)**	**Duration (weeks)**	**Intervention**	**Outcomes**	**Significant findings associated with exercise only**
			AER + RX (no description RX)	*Anthropometric* BW, WHR, BF%, lean body mass *Menstrual cyclicity/ reproductive* Menstrual status, ovulation *Other measurements* Caloric intake/ 24 hrs, steps/d	
Curi et al., 2012, [86] RCT	E = 40 C = 27	24	a. Metformin (850 mg) 2× day b. Lifestyle and diet (carb 50%, fat 30%, protein 20%), 30 min walk, 3 RX (squats, pushups, sit-ups)	*Hemotological* Fasting blood glucose, insulin, gonadotropins, E_2, total T, A, DHEA-S, tg, C *Anthropometric* BMI, WC *Menstrual cyclicity/ reproductive* Menstrual cycle index	BMI, WC, MCI
Almenning et al., 2015, [80] RCT	E = 31 C = 25	10	3× wk. (1× supervised) a. RT- 8 dynamic strength drills- 75% 1RM, 3×10. b. HITT-2× sessions (4×4 min 90–95% HR_{max}, and 3 min moderate intensity 70% HR_{max}) 1 session (10× 1 min max intensity, 1 min rest/very low activity). Self-selected (treadmill, walking/running/ cycling) c. Control	*Hemotological* IR (HOMA-IR), Glucose, C, HDL, LDL, tg, CRP. Insulin, adiponectin, leptin, T, homocysteine, AMH, FAI, SHBG, DHEA-S *Cardiorespiratory* VO_{2max} *Hemodynamic* Heart rate recovery *Anthropometric* BW, WC, FM, VF, FFM, BF% *Menstrual cyclicity/ reproductive* menstrual frequency *Other measurements* Endothelial vasodilation (FMD)	HOMA-IR, HDL, AMH, endothelial function, BF%
Turan et al., 2015, [83] RCT	E = 32 C = 30	8	3× wk. 8 weeks. a. AER + RX (50–60 min) AER- Step 5–20 min (Borg 10–15) RX-Elastic band 15 reps each (intensity 5–6	*Hemotological* FSH, LH, FSH, E2, Total T, fT, HDL, LDL, tg, Total cholesterol, fasting glucose, fasting insulin, HOMA *Cardiorespiratory*	WC, HC, DBP, RR, VO_{2max}, LDL, total cholesterol, fasting glucose, HOMA, mean menstrual cycle interval

Mixed interventions (aerobic and/or resistance)

Author, Study design	N enrolled (E) & completed (C)	Duration (weeks)	Intervention	Outcomes	Significant findings associated with exercise only
			somewhat intense) a. Control	VO_{2max} *Hemodynamic* SBP, DBP, HR, RR *Anthropometric* BMI, WC, HC *Other measurements* IPAQ	
Nasiri et al., 2022 [81], RCT	E = 45 C = 45	8	a. HITT-4×30 s 100% maximum speed, 4×30 s active recovery, 5 min passive recovery. b. COM- 3× wk, RX 3×10–16 repetitions (50–70% 1RM) and AER – running 60–70% HR_{max} c. Usual care	*Cardiorespiratory* VO_{2max} *Anthropometric* BMI, WHR, Weight, BF%, VAT	BMI, WHR, BF%, VAT, VO_{2max}
Rao et al., 2022, [82] RCT	E = 50 C = 40	12	a. HITT-3× treadmill (4×4 at 90–95% HR_{max}, and 3 min moderate intensity (70% HR_{max})- 45 min session, total duration HITT 25 min b. RX-3× wk., 60–70% 1RM 3×10	*Hemotological* T *Anthropometric* BMI, BF% *Questionnaire* IPAQ	BMI (both groups), T, BF% and IPAQ (more in HITT)

Resistance training interventions

Author, Study design	N enrolled & completed	Duration	Intervention	Outcomes	Findings ($P < 0.005$)
Lara et al., 2015, [89] Ramos et al., 2016, [90] Kogure et al. 2019, [92] Kogure et al., 2018 [93], 2016 [94], Miranda-Furtado et al., 2015 [95] NRCT	E = 115 C = 94 *(43 PCOS and 51 healthy controls)*	16	RX- 2 wks adaptation RX 3× wk (upper and lower body exercises)- 4 microcycles (4 weeks each) 1st macrocycle- 3×15 (60%, 65%, 70%, 65%) 2nd macrocycle- 3×12 (65%, 70%, 75%, 70%) 3rd macrocycle-3×10 (70%, 75%, 80%, 75%) 4th macrocycle 3×8 (75%, 80%, 85%, and 80%)	*Hemotological* T, A, Glucose, Insulin, HOMA-IR, LH, FSH, E_2, SHBG, FAI, 17-OHP, homocysteine *Anthropometric* Height, BW, BMI, WC, lean muscle mass (total LM, trunk LM, BF%, LM/height^2), arm muscle area (cm), thigh	T, A, SHBG, fasting glucose, total LM, Trunk LM, BF%, LM/height^2, WC, WHR Total score (FSFI), HADS, SF-36 (functional capacity), arm muscle area, maximum strength (bench press, leg press,

Resistance training interventions					
Author, Study design	**N enrolled & completed**	**Duration**	**Intervention**	**Outcomes**	**Findings (P < 0.005)**
				muscle area (cm) *Questionnaire* PARQ, FSFI, HADS, SF-36 *Other measurement* Telomere content	leg extension), telomere content
Vizza et al., 2006, [17] RCT	E = 15 C = 10	12	a. RX 2× wk. supervised (3×12 upper/ lower body) and 2× unsupervised sessions at home b. Control	*Hemotological* HOMA-2, CRP, T, SHBG, FAI, HbA1c, fasting glucose, fasting insulin *Anthropometric* Height, BW, BMI, WC, HC, WHR, FM, LM, FFM, BF% *Hemodynamic* SBP, DBP *Questionnaire* PCOSQ, SF-36, DASS-21, Exercise self-efficacy scale *Menstrual cyclicity/ reproductive* Menstrual cyclicity *Functional* Isometric maximum voluntary contraction upper and lower body *Other measurements* Feasibility outcomes (recruitment and attrition, adherence, adverse events, completion assessments)	BW, BMI, WC, LM, FFM, HbA1c, fasting glucose, trend upper body strength, lower body strength, PCOSQ (emotions, weight, infertility problems), SF-36 (physical functioning, vitality, social functioning, role emotional, mental health), DASS-21, exercise self efficacy
Ribeiro et al. 2016, [47] case control	E = 53 *(27 PCOS and 26 control)*	16	RX 70% 1RM, 12 repetitions, (upper and lower body exercises)-mesocycles (4wk each) Wk 1–3: 3× wk., intensity increased 5% wk.	*Hemotological* T, A, T/A ratio, SHBG, FAI, fasting glucose, fasting insulin, HOMA-IR *Anthropometric*	N.S between groups (PCOS did show within group LF, HF, LH/HF ratio)

Resistance training interventions					
Author, Study design	**N enrolled & completed**	**Duration**	**Intervention**	**Outcomes**	**Findings (P < 0.005)**
			Wk 4: 2× wk, intensity decreased 5%	Weight, BMI, BF% *Hemodynamic* HR, SBP, DBP, MBP, HRV	
Saremi et al., 2016 [96], RCT	E = 33 C = 31	8	a. RX and placebo b. RX and calcium supplement c. Control RX 3× wk. 1–2 sets 5–20 reps at 40–60% 1RM (upper and lower body)	*Hemotological* Total C, Tg, LDL, HDL, HOMA-IR, fasting insulin, fasting glucose *Anthropometric* BW *Strength* chest press and leg press	Fasting insulin, fasting blood glucose, tg, cholesterol, LDL, HDL, HOMA-IR, upper/lower body strength, weight. AMH (combined only)
Ramos et al., 2016, [90] NRCT	E = 94 C = 94 *(43 PCOS and 51 healthy controls)*	16	RX: 3×10, %1RM (upper and lower body exercises) 4× microcycles 4 weeks each (60%, 65%, 70%, 75%)	*Hemotological* T, A, glucose, insulin, HOMA-IR *Anthropometric* WC, BMI, Weight *Questionnaire* SF-36	T (PCOS and control), A (PCOS), WC (PCOS), SF-36 (functional capacity), vitality, social aspects, mental health (healthy controls)
Zhang et al., 2017, [88] RCT	E = 101 C = 101	24	a. Metformin (500 mg 3× day) and clomiphene (2× 50–100)- 5 consecutive days for 3 consecutive menstrual cycles b. Lifestyle (strengthening, 30 min each and stopped when patients began to sweat)	*Hemotological* LH, T, LH/FSH, fasting insulin, TG *Anthropometric* WHR, BMI, BW *Menstrual cyclicity/ reproductive* Left ovarian volume, right ovarian volume, endometrial thickness, menstrual recovery rate, ovulation rate, pregnancy rate	BW, BMI, LH, T, LH/FSH, fasting insulin, TG, left/ right ovarian volumes, menstrual recovery, ovulation and pregnancy rate
Hosseini et al., 2019, [97] RCT	E = 60 C = 60	8	a. Control b. Water training (upper/lower trunk strength training) 3×12, 60 min c. RX 30 min 40–70% RM (does	*Hemotological* AMH *Anthropometric* BW	AMH (training in water with vit D and Vit D)

Resistance training interventions					
Author, Study design	**N enrolled & completed**	**Duration**	**Intervention**	**Outcomes**	**Findings ($P < 0.005$)**
			not list exercises) d. VitD e. VitD and water training f. Land training and VitD		
Saeed et al., 2022, [98] case control	E = 143 C = 79 *(PCOS and 64 non PCOS)*	8	RX 3×10, %1RM Upper and Lower body exercises	*Hemotological* Fasting glucose, fasting insulin, T, A *Anthropometric* Height, BMI, WC *Questionnaire* PARQ, SF-36	SF-36 (role functional, role physical, pain, energy)
Aqdas et al., 2022, [87] NRCT	E = 28 A = 28	12	Not described	*Hemotological* Total C, HDL, LDL, Tg, *Anthropometric* BMI	BMI, Total C, HDL, LDL, Tg

Abbreviations: T, testosterone; SHBG, sex hormone binding globulin; E_2, estradiol; LH, lutenizing hormone; FSH, follicle stimulating hormone; P, progesterone; DHEA-S, dehydroepiandrosterone; A, Androstenedione; 17-OHP, 17-Hydroxyprogesterone; FAI, free androgen index; TSH, thyroid stimulating hormone; PDG, pregnanediol-3-glucoronide; C, cholesterol; TC, total cholesterol; Tg, triglycerides; LDL, low density lipoprotein; HDL, high density lipoprotein; HOMA-IR, homeostatic model assessment insulin resistance; QUICKI, quantitative insulin-sensitivity check index; IGF-1, insulin growth factor; T_4, thyroxine; CRP, C-reactive protein; WBC, white blood cells; BMI, body mass index; BF%, body fat percentage; FM, fat mass; FFM, fat free mass; AbFm, abdominal fat mass; WC, waist circumference; WHR, waist to hip ratio; HC, hip circumference; SO2S, sum of 2 skinfolds; REE, resting energy expenditure; SBP, systolic blood pressure; DBP, diastolic blood pressure; IPAQ, International physical activity questionnaire; HbA1c- glycated hemoglobin; HR, heart rate; HRR, heart rate reserve; VO_{2max}, maximal oxygen consumption; VO_{2AT}, maximal oxygen consumption at anaerobic threshold; VE/VCO_{2slope}, minute ventilation-carbon dioxide production; AER+RX, aerobic plus resistance; RCT, randomized control trial; RM, repetition maximum; NRCT, non randomized control trial; BW, body weight; FFA, free fatty acid; BMD, bone mineral density; PCOSQ, Polycystic Ovary Syndrome Questionnaire; E1, estrone; E1-s, E1 sulphate; 5-DIOL, 5-androstene-3; ADT-G, androsterone glucuronide; 3G, androstane-3; 17G, 17-diol-17 glucuronide; BSA-S, Brief Scale for Anxiety; SF-36, Short form-36; NS, not significant; NEFA, non, esterified free fatty acids; RBC, red blood cell; HTC, hematocrit; MCV, mean corpuscular volume; MCH, mean corpuscular hemoglobin; MCHC, mean corpuscular hemoglobin concentration; PTL, platelets total level; TBW, total body water; BMR, basal metabolic rate; HRV, heart rate variability; CAT, continuous aerobic training; IAT, intermittent aerobic training; FSRI, Female sexual function index; FRS, figure rating scale; HITT, high intensity interval training; GGT, gamma-glutamyl transferase; ALT, alanine aminotransferase; A/P, Atherogenic index of plasma; TS/C, testosterone to cortisol ratio; VAT, visceral adipose tissue; VAI, visceral adiposity index; CES-D, Center for Epidemiologic Studies Depression Scale; STAI, State–Trait Anxiety Inventory; PSS, perceived stress scale; ACE, adverse childhood experience; TSST, Trier Social stress test; DASS-21, depression anxiety and stress score; IFG, impaired fasting glucose; RER, respiratory exchange ratio; PLT, platelets total level; GDR, glucose disposal rate; IL-6, interleukin-6.

Table 2.
Summary exercise studies (aerobic and resistance, and resistance training in isolation).

supervised training [17, 80], 40–45% for home-based calisthenics training [17], or 60% overall for both supervised and home-based calisthenics training [17]. In addition, similar to the aerobic training studies, dropout rates were also not always reported across these studies. Of the studies that reported this, this ranged between 10%–50%, where a higher drop out rate was reported in studies that included a dietary restriction [79, 85].

Characteristics (e.g., age and BMI) were also similar as per the aerobic studies only (Section 2.1), and in addition, most studies also had similar exclusion criteria as per the aerobic training studies. Further, similar to the aerobic training studies, limited studies included PCOS participants with a BMI < 25.0 kg/m^2 [83], nor did they report on ethnicity outcomes [17, 78–82, 84–86]. Furthermore, other baseline characteristics that were also not included in the aerobic training studies (e.g., family history, co morbidities, pain perception, sleep apnea, previous pregnancy etc.) were also not reported in these studies. Although it may be possible that some studies have reported these as supplementary materials, or this information may not be available due to the exclusion criteria across studies.

The benefits of resistance training interventions in PCOS ranged from improved body composition (e.g., reduced waist circumference, hip circumference, BMI, body weight, and improved lean muscle mass), improved insulin sensitivity and menstrual cyclicity, and quality of life (such as anxiety, depression). In addition, for studies that included normal weight PCOS, possible benefits following a resistance training intervention may include changes in body composition (e.g., waist circumference, hip circumference), shorter menstrual cycle intervals, and hematological changes (e.g., cholesterol).

A detailed list of outcomes for each of these studies and their findings are provided in **Table 2**.

2.3 Conclusion and future directions for research

A large number of exercise interventions have been evaluated in PCOS, and benefits are noted across aerobic, moderate and high intensity, lifestyle and resistance training interventions. Variability was noted across studies in terms of reporting baseline characteristics of PCOS, description of interventions, as well as reporting of co-interventions. Overall, while the benefits of exercise were noted across interventions, higher dropout rates are often noted in women with PCOS, which may affect overall study findings. Although this was not reported across all studies, future studies should also continue to report on both drop out and/or compliance rates across all interventions.

These findings will allow future research to determine as to which interventions would require further strategies for women with PCOS in order to improve overall adherence and compliance. Possible strategies could include the measurement of exercise self-efficacy at baseline to determine predictors of long-term adherence, as well as include a long-term follow-up component to better understand if additional barriers are noted for women with PCOS to adopt the lifestyle behavior change. Further, focus groups and/or interviews with study participants could also be incorporated, and their feedback could be integrated into the intervention to address for any other barriers. Furthermore, studies may also consider and test other methods of delivering the exercise interventions to improve compliance such as Telehealth, home based visits and/or online/zoom.

These strategies could also be incorporated for participants in the cultural and linguistically diverse community (CALD) and will allow researchers to better understand reasons for non-compliance and/or higher drop out which was reported in a few studies. This could also be coupled with further reporting of other baseline characteristics in PCOS to determine if there are any other contributing factors that may result in non-compliance, for example, physical and/or psychological, or whether participants may be using other co-interventions outside of the study that may be more effective as opposed to the intervention. Further, studies should also look to report other ethnicity measures (e.g., Ancestry, as well as those with limited English language proficiency), to better understand ethnic groups that may be at at risk of poorer outcomes and require ongoing management.

While the majority of studies included PCOS women with a BMI >25.0 kg/m^2, most studies excluded participants with a history of conditions such as cardiovascular disease, metabolic syndrome, glucose intolerance etc. As women with PCOS are at an elevated risk for the development of these conditions, future studies should look to include these participants with a number of co-morbidities, in order to determine for differences between controls for both baseline characteristics, as well as overall response to exercise. In addition, further studies should also look to report on other outcomes such as previous pregnancies and/or whether they were diagnosed with previous gestational diabetes in pregnancy, in order to understand as to whether it may lead to changes in the metabolic profile and/or symptomology of PCOS versus non pregnant participants, or whether it may lead to differences in the response rate to exercise.

Also, limited studies included PCOS women with a BMI <25.0 kg/m^2, and further studies are warranted to better understand both the baseline characteristics in this group (physical and psychological) and the benefits of exercise. Studies may also look to incorporate focus groups to better understand the lived experience in this group, and these findings could enable both the researchers and clinicians to incorporate recommendations to improve overall management and tailor interventions appropriately.

Conflict of interest

The author declares no conflict of interest.

Notes/thanks/other declarations

A big thankyou to my family (Raffaele, Rosa, Angela, Laura, Maurizio and Neil), niece and nephews (Chloe, Ollie, Patrick) for their ongoing support to allow me to continue contributing to important research. Also, to close friends (Claudia, Jodie, Maureen, Brunelle, Nancy, Mereani, Michelle, Lana, Kathy, Joanna, Sarah, Chantay) and supervisors at my current role (Christina and Sharon), I am forever thankful for your support, mentorship, feedback, and encouragement for me to work on this chapter and to contribute to this important work.

Author details

Lisa Vizza
University of Sydney, Sydney, Australia

*Address all correspondence to: lisavizza@sydney.edu.au; lisavizza@hotmail.com

References

[1] March WA, Moore VM, Willson KJ, Phillips DI, Norman RJ, Davies MJ. The prevalence of polycystic ovary syndrome in a community sample assessed under contrasting diagnostic criteria. Human Reproduction. 2010;**25**(2):544-551. DOI: 10.1093/humrep/dep399

[2] Revised 2003 consensus on diagnostic criteria and long-term health risks related to polycystic ovary syndrome. Fertility and Sterility. 2004;**81**(1):19-25. DOI: 10.1093/humrep/deh098

[3] Escobar-Morreale HF. Polycystic ovary syndrome: Definition, aetiology, diagnosis and treatment. Nature Reviews. Endocrinology. 2018;**14**(5): 270-284. DOI: 10.1038/nrendo.2018.24

[4] Hoeger KM, Dokras A, Piltonen T. Update on PCOS: Consequences, challenges, and guiding treatment. The Journal of Clinical Endocrinology & Metabolism. 2021;**106**(3):e1071-e1e83. DOI: 10.1210/clinem/dgaa839

[5] Stepto NK, Cassar S, Joham AE, Hutchison SK, Harrison CL, Goldstein RF, et al. Women with polycystic ovary syndrome have intrinsic insulin resistance on euglycaemic–hyperinsulaemic clamp. Human Reproduction. 2013;**28**(3):777-784. DOI: 10.1093/humrep/des463

[6] Cassar S, Misso ML, Hopkins WG, Shaw CS, Teede HJ, Stepto NK. Insulin resistance in polycystic ovary syndrome: A systematic review and meta-analysis of euglycaemic–hyperinsulinaemic clamp studies. Human Reproduction. 2016;**31**(11):2619-2631. DOI: 10.1093/humrep/dew243

[7] Azziz R, Carmina E, Dewailly D, Diamanti-Kandarakis E, Escobar-Morreale HF, Futterweit W, et al. The androgen excess and PCOS society criteria for the polycystic ovary syndrome: The complete task force report. Fertility and Sterility. 2009; **91**(2):456-488. DOI: 10.1016/j.fertnstert.2008.06.035

[8] Dunaif A, Segal KR, Shelley DR, Green G, Dobrjansky A, Licholai T. Evidence for distinctive and intrinsic defects in insulin action in polycystic ovary syndrome. Diabetes. 1992;**41**(10): 1257-1266. DOI: 10.2337/diab.41.10.1257

[9] Melo AS, Ferriani RA, Navarro PA. Treatment of infertility in women with polycystic ovary syndrome: Approach to clinical practice. Clinics (São Paulo, Brazil). 2015;**70**(11):765-769. DOI: 10.6061/clinics/2015(11)09

[10] Bloomgarden ZT. Second world congress on the insulin resistance syndrome: Insulin resistance syndrome and nonalcoholic fatty liver disease. Diabetes Care. 2005;**28**(6):1518. DOI: 10.2337/diacare.28.6.1518

[11] Lin H, Liu M, Zhong D, Ng EHY, Liu J, Li J, et al. The prevalence and factors associated with anxiety-like and depression-like behaviors in women with polycystic ovary syndrome. Frontiers in Psychiatry. 2021;**12**:709674. DOI: 10.3389/fpsyt.2021.709674

[12] Barnard L, Ferriday D, Guenther N, Strauss B, Balen AH, Dye L. Quality of life and psychological well being in polycystic ovary syndrome. Human Reproduction. 2007;**22**(8):2279-2286. DOI: 10.1093/humrep/dem108

[13] Barry JA, Kuczmierczyk AR, Hardiman PJ. Anxiety and depression in polycystic ovary syndrome: A systematic review and meta-analysis. Human

Reproduction. 2011;**26**(9):2442-2451. DOI: 10.1093/humrep/der197

[14] Teede HJ, Misso ML, Deeks AA, Moran LJ, Stuckey BG, Wong JL, et al. Assessment and management of polycystic ovary syndrome: Summary of an evidence-based guideline. The Medical Journal of Australia. 2011; **195**(6):S65. DOI: 10.5694/mja11.10915

[15] Ibañez J, Izquierdo M, Ia A, Forga L, Larrión JL, García-Unciti M, et al. Twice-weekly progressive resistance training decreases abdominal fat and improves insulin sensitivity in older men with type 2 diabetes. Diabetes Care. 2005;**28**(3): 662-667. DOI: 10.2337/diacare.28.3.662

[16] Qadir R, Sculthorpe NF, Todd T, Brown EC. Effectiveness of resistance training and associated program characteristics in patients at risk for type 2 diabetes: A systematic review and meta-analysis. Sports Medicine – Open. 2021;**7**(1):38. DOI: 10.1186/s40798-021-00321-x

[17] Vizza L, Smith CA, Swaraj S, Agho K, Cheema BS. The feasibility of progressive resistance training in women with polycystic ovary syndrome: A pilot randomized controlled trial. BMC Sports Science, Medicine and Rehabilitation. 2016;**8**:14. DOI: 10.1186/s13102-016-0039-8

[18] Misso M. International evidence-based guideline for the assessment and management of polycystic ovary syndrome 2018. National Health and Medical Research Council (NHMRC) on. 2018;2. Available from: https://www.monash.edu/__data/assets/pdf_file/0004/1412644/PCOS_Evidence-Based-Guidelines_20181009.pdf

[19] American College of Sports Medicine. ACSM's guidelines for exercise testing and prescription. USA: Lippincott Williams & Wilkins; 2013

[20] Abazar E, Taghian F, Mardanian F, Forozandeh D. Effects of aerobic exercise on plasma lipoproteins in overweight and obese women with polycystic ovary syndrome. Advanced Biomedical Research. 2015;**2005**:4. DOI: 10.4103/2277-9175.153892

[21] Al-Eisa E, Gabr SA, Alghadir AH. Effects of supervised aerobic training on the levels of anti-Mullerian hormone and adiposity measures in women with normo-ovulatory and polycystic ovary syndrome. JPMA The Journal of the Pakistan Medical Association. 2017; **67**(4):499-507

[22] Covington JD, Bajpeyi S, Moro C, Tchoukalova YD, Ebenezer PJ, Burk DH, et al. Potential effects of aerobic exercise on the expression of perilipin 3 in the adipose tissue of women with polycystic ovary syndrome: A pilot study. European Journal of Endocrinology. 2015;**172**(1): 47-58. DOI: 10.1530/EJE-14-0492

[23] Elbandrawy A, Yousef A, Morgan E, Ewais N, Eid M, Elkholi S, et al. Effect of aerobic exercise on inflammatory markers in polycystic ovary syndrome: A randomized controlled trial. European Review for Medical & Pharmacological Sciences. 2022;**26**(10):3506-3513. DOI: 10.26355/eurrev_202205_28845

[24] Giallauria F, Orio F, Palomba S, Lombardi G, Colao A, Vigorito C. Cardiovascular risk in women with polycystic ovary syndrome. Journal of Cardiovascular Medicine. 2008;**9**(10): 987-992. DOI: 10.2459/JCM.0b013e32830b58d4

[25] Kostrzewa-Nowak D, Nowak R, Jastrzębski Z, Zarębska A, Bichowska M, Drobnik-Kozakiewicz I, et al. Effect of 12-week-long aerobic training

programme on body composition, aerobic capacity, complete blood count and blood lipid profile among young women. Biochemia Medica. 2015;**25**(1): 103-113. DOI: 10.11613/BM.2015.013

[26] Moro C, Pasarica M, Elkind-Hirsch K, Redman LM. Aerobic exercise training improves atrial natriuretic peptide and catecholamine-mediated lipolysis in obese women with polycystic ovary syndrome. The Journal of Clinical Endocrinology & Metabolism. 2009; **94**(7):2579-2586. DOI: 10.1210/jc.2009-0051

[27] Palomba S, Giallauria F, Falbo A, Russo T, Oppedisano R, Tolino A, et al. Structured exercise training programme versus hypocaloric hyperproteic diet in obese polycystic ovary syndrome patients with anovulatory infertility: A 24-week pilot study. Human Reproduction. 2008;**23**(3):642-650. DOI: 10.1093/humrep/dem391

[28] Ramanjaneya M, Abdalhakam I, Bettahi I, Bensila M, Jerobin J, Aye MM, et al. Effect of moderate aerobic exercise on complement activation pathways in polycystic ovary syndrome women. Frontiers in Endocrinology. 2022;**12**: 740703. DOI: 10.3389/fendo.2021.740703

[29] Vigorito C, Giallauria F, Palomba S, Cascella T, Manguso F, Lucci R, et al. Beneficial effects of a three-month structured exercise training program on cardiopulmonary functional capacity in young women with polycystic ovary syndrome. The Journal of Clinical Endocrinology & Metabolism. 2007; **92**(4):1379-1384. DOI: 10.1210/jc.2006-2794

[30] Jedel E, Labrie F, Odén A, Holm G, Nilsson L, Janson PO, et al. Impact of electro-acupuncture and physical exercise on hyperandrogenism and oligo/amenorrhea in women with polycystic ovary syndrome: A randomized controlled trial. American Journal of Physiology. Endocrinology and Metabolism. 2011;**300**(1):E37-E45. DOI: 10.1152/ajpendo.00495.2010

[31] Stener-Victorin E, Holm G, Janson PO, Gustafson D, Waern M. Acupuncture and physical exercise for affective symptoms and health-related quality of life in polycystic ovary syndrome: Secondary analysis from a randomized controlled trial. BMC Complementary and Alternative Medicine. 2013;**13**(1):1-8. DOI: 10.1186/1472-6882-13-131

[32] Brown AJ, Setji TL, Sanders LL, Lowry KP, Otvos JD, Kraus WE, et al. Effects of exercise on lipoprotein particles in women with polycystic ovary syndrome. Medicine and Science in Sports and Exercise. 2009;**41**(3):497. DOI: 10.1249/MSS.0b013e31818c6c0c

[33] Costa EC, DE Sá JCF, Stepto NK, Costa IBB, Farias-Junior LF, Moreira SDNT, et al. Aerobic Training Improves Quality of Life in Women with Polycystic Ovary Syndrome. Medicine & Science in Sports & Exercise. Jul 2018;**50** (7):1357-1366. DOI: 10.1249/MSS.0000000000001579. PMID: 29443823

[34] Randeva HS, Lewandowski KC, Jz D, Brooke-Wavell K, O'Callaghan C, Czupryniak L, et al. Exercise decreases plasma total homocysteine in overweight young women with polycystic ovary syndrome. The Journal of Clinical Endocrinology & Metabolism. 2002; **87**(10):4496-4501. DOI: 10.1210/jc.2001-012056

[35] Sa JC, Costa EC, da Silva E, Tamburús NY, Porta A, Medeiros LF, et al. Aerobic exercise improves cardiac autonomic modulation in women with polycystic ovary syndrome.

International Journal of Cardiology. 2016;**202**:356-361. DOI: 10.1016/j.ijcard.2015.09.031

[36] Stener-Victorin E, Jedel E, Janson PO, Sverrisdottir YB. Low-frequency electroacupuncture and physical exercise decrease high muscle sympathetic nerve activity in polycystic ovary syndrome. American Journal of Physiology-Regulatory, Integrative and Comparative Physiology. 2009;**2009**: R387-R395. DOI: 10.1152/ajpregu.00197.2009

[37] Benham JL, Booth JE, Corenblum B, Doucette S, Friedenreich CM, Rabi DM, et al. Exercise training and reproductive outcomes in women with polycystic ovary syndrome: A pilot randomized controlled trial. Clinical Endocrinology. 2021;**95**(2):332-343. DOI: 10.1111/cen.14452

[38] Faryadian B, Tadibi V, Behpour N. Effect of 12-week high intensity interval training program on C-reactive protein and insulin resistance in women with polycystic ovary syndrome. Journal of Clinical & Diagnostic Research. 2019;**13**(9):CC01-CC04. DOI: 10.7860/JCDR/2019/41203.13106

[39] Gaeini A, Satarifard S, Mohamadi F, Choobineh S. The effect of 12 weeks aerobic exercise on DHEAso4, 17OH-Progestron concentrations, number of follicles and menstrual condition of women with PCOS. Hormozgan Medical Journal. 2021;**18**(4):298-305

[40] Harrison CL, Stepto NK, Hutchison SK, Teede HJ. The impact of intensified exercise training on insulin resistance and fitness in overweight and obese women with and without polycystic ovary syndrome. Clinical Endocrinology. 2012;**76**(3):351-357. DOI: 10.1111/j.1365-2265.2011.04160.x

[41] Hutchison SK, Stepto NK, Harrison CL, Moran LJ, Strauss BJ, Teede HJ. Effects of exercise on insulin resistance and body composition in overweight and obese women with and without polycystic ovary syndrome. The Journal of Clinical Endocrinology & Metabolism. 2011;**96**(1):E48-E56. DOI: 10.1210/jc.2010-0828

[42] Hutchison SK, Teede HJ, Rachoń D, Harrison CL, Strauss BJ, Stepto NK. Effect of exercise training on insulin sensitivity, mitochondria and computed tomography muscle attenuation in overweight women with and without polycystic ovary syndrome. Diabetologia. 2012;**55**:1424-1434. DOI: 10.1007/s00125-011-2442-8

[43] Kogure GS, Lopes IP, Ribeiro VB, Mendes MC, Kodato S, Furtado CLM, et al. The effects of aerobic physical exercises on body image among women with polycystic ovary syndrome. Journal of Affective Disorders. 2020;**262**: 350-358. DOI: 10.1016/j.jad.2019.11.025

[44] Lopes IP, Ribeiro VB, Reis RM, Silva RC, Dutra de Souza HC, Kogure GS, et al. Comparison of the effect of intermittent and continuous aerobic physical training on sexual function of women with polycystic ovary syndrome: Randomized controlled trial. The Journal of Sexual Medicine. 2018;**15**(11):1609-1619. DOI: 10.1016/j.jsxm.2018.09.002

[45] Mohammadi S, Monazzami A, Alavimilani S. Effects of eight-week high-intensity interval training on some metabolic, hormonal and cardiovascular indices in women with PCOS: A randomized controlled trail. BMC Sports Science, Medicine and Rehabilitation. 2023;**15**(1):47. DOI: 10.1186/s13102-023-00653-z

[46] Moran LJ, Harrison CL, Hutchison SK, Stepto N, Strauss BJ,

Teede HJ. Exercise decreases anti-Müllerian hormone in anovulatory overweight women with polycystic ovary syndrome–a pilot study. Hormone and Metabolic Research. 2011;**2011**: 977-979. DOI: 10.1055/s-0031-1291208

[47] Ribeiro VB, Lopes IP, Dos Reis RM, Silva RC, Mendes MC, Melo AS, et al. Continuous versus intermittent aerobic exercise in the improvement of quality of life for women with polycystic ovary syndrome: A randomized controlled trial. Journal of Health Psychology. 2021; **26**(9):1307-1317. DOI: 10.1177/1359105319869806

[48] Roessler KK, Birkebaek C, Ravn P, Andersen MS, Glintborg D. Effects of exercise and group counselling on body composition and VO 2max in overweight women with polycystic ovary syndrome. Acta obstetricia et Gynecologica Scandinavica. 2013;**92**(3):272-277. DOI: 10.1111/aogs.12064

[49] Scott D, Harrison CL, Hutchison S, De Courten B, Stepto NK. Exploring factors related to changes in body composition, insulin sensitivity and aerobic capacity in response to a 12-week exercise intervention in overweight and obese women with and without polycystic ovary syndrome. PLoS One. 2017;**12**(8):e0182412. DOI: 10.1371/journal.pone.0182412

[50] Arentz S, Smith CA, Abbott J, Fahey P, Cheema BS, Bensoussan A. Combined lifestyle and herbal medicine in overweight women with polycystic ovary syndrome (PCOS): A randomized controlled trial. Phytotherapy Research. 2017;**31**(9):1330-1340. DOI: 10.1002/ptr.5858

[51] Cooney LG, Milman LW, Hantsoo L, Kornfield S, Sammel MD, Allison KC, et al. Cognitive-behavioral therapy improves weight loss and quality of life in women with polycystic ovary syndrome: A pilot randomized clinical trial. Fertility and Sterility. 2018;**110**(1):161-171. DOI: 10.1016/j.fertnstert.2018.03.028

[52] De Frène V, Verhofstadt L, Lammertyn J, Stuyver I, Buysse A, De Sutter P. Quality of life and body mass index in overweight adult women with polycystic ovary syndrome during a lifestyle modification program. Journal of Obstetric, Gynecologic, and Neonatal Nursing. 2015;**44**(5):587-599. DOI: 10.1111/1552-6909.12739

[53] Dokras A, Sarwer DB, Allison KC, Milman L, Kris-Etherton PM, Kunselman AR, et al. Weight loss and lowering androgens predict improvements in health-related quality of life in women with PCOS. The Journal of Clinical Endocrinology & Metabolism. 2016;**101**(8):2966-2974. DOI: 10.1210/jc.2016-1896

[54] Hoeger KM, Kochman L, Wixom N, Craig K, Miller RK, Guzick DS. A randomized, 48-week, placebo-controlled trial of intensive lifestyle modification and/or metformin therapy in overweight women with polycystic ovary syndrome: A pilot study. Fertility and Sterility. 2004;**82**(2):421-429. DOI: 10.1016/j.fertnstert.2004.02.104

[55] Konopka AR, Asante A, Lanza IR, Robinson MM, Johnson ML, Dalla Man C, et al. Defects in mitochondrial efficiency and H2O2 emissions in obese women are restored to a lean phenotype with aerobic exercise training. Diabetes. 2015;**64**(6):2104-2115. DOI: 10.2337/db14-1701

[56] Ladson G, Dodson WC, Sweet SD, Archibong AE, Kunselman AR, Demers LM, et al. The effects of metformin with lifestyle therapy in polycystic ovary syndrome: A randomized double-blind study. Fertility

and Sterility. 2011;**95**(3):1059-1066. DOI: 10.1016/j.fertnstert.2010.12.002

[57] Legro RS, Dodson WC, Kris-Etherton PM, Kunselman AR, Stetter CM, Williams NI, et al. Randomized controlled trial of preconception interventions in infertile women with polycystic ovary syndrome. The Journal of Clinical Endocrinology and Metabolism. 2015;**100**(11): 4048-4058. DOI: 10.1210/jc.2015-2778

[58] Mahoney D. Lifestyle modification intervention among infertile overweight and obese women with polycystic ovary syndrome. Journal of the American Association of Nurse Practitioners. 2014; **26**(6):301-308. DOI: 10.1002/2327-6924.12073

[59] Manteghi G, Shahraki Z, Moghadam MN, Ghanbarpour MH. Pregnancy outcome in PCOS patients: The effects of letrozol combined with exercise. Journal für Klinische Endokrinologie und Stoffwechsel. 2021; **14**(3):128-132. DOI: 10.1007/s41969-021-00142-z

[60] Nagelberg J, Burks H, Mucowski S, Shoupe D. The effect of home exercise on ovulation induction using clomiphene citrate in overweight underserved women with polycystic ovarian syndrome. Contraception and Reproductive Medicine. 2016;**1**(1):14. DOI: 10.1186/s40834-016-0025-2

[61] Pandit U, Singh M, Ranjan R, Gupta V. The effect of exercise training on body composition, insulin resistance and high sensitivity C-reactive protein (Hs-CRP) in women with polycystic ovary syndrome: A Pilot Study From North India. Cureus. 2022;**14**(4):1-7, e23994. DOI: 10.7759/cureus.23994

[62] Liao LM, Nesic J, Chadwick PM, Brooke-Wavell K, Prelevic GM. Exercise and body image distress in overweight and obese women with polycystic ovary syndrome: A pilot investigation. Gynecological Endocrinology. 2008; **24**(10):555-561. DOI: 10.1080/09513590802288226

[63] Orio F, Muscogiuri G, Giallauria F, Savastano S, Bottiglieri P, Tafuri D, et al. Oral contraceptives versus physical exercise on cardiovascular and metabolic risk factors in women with polycystic ovary syndrome: A randomized controlled trial. Clinical Endocrinology. 2016;**85**(5):764-771. DOI: 10.1111/cen.13112

[64] Gilani N, Zamani Rad F, Ebrahimi M, Haghshenas R. Effect of eight weeks endurance training on ovarian androgens in women with polycystic ovary syndrome: Application of multivariate longitudinal models. International Journal of Applied Exercise Physiology. 2019;**8**(2):657-672

[65] McBreairty LE, Kazemi M, Chilibeck PD, Gordon JJ, Chizen DR, Zello GA. Effect of a pulse-based diet and aerobic exercise on bone measures and body composition in women with polycystic ovary syndrome: A randomized controlled trial. Bone Reports. 2020;**12**:100248. DOI: 10.1016/j.bonr.2020.100248

[66] Kazemi M, Pierson RA, McBreairty LE, Chilibeck PD, Zello GA, Chizen DR. A randomized controlled trial of a lifestyle intervention with longitudinal follow-up on ovarian dysmorphology in women with polycystic ovary syndrome. Clinical Endocrinology. 2020;**92**(6):525-535. DOI: 10.1111/cen.14179

[67] Wu X, Wu H, Sun W, Wang C. Improvement of anti-Müllerian hormone and oxidative stress through regular exercise in Chinese women with

polycystic ovary syndrome. Hormones. 2021;**20**(2):339-345. DOI: 10.1007/s42000-020-00233-7

[68] Philbois SV, Ribeiro VB, Tank J, Dos Reis RM, Gerlach DA, Souza HCD. Cardiovascular autonomic modulation differences between moderate-intensity continuous and high-intensity interval aerobic training in women with PCOS: A randomized trial. Front Endocrinology (Lausanne). 2022;**13**:1024844. DOI: 10.3389/fendo.2022.1024844

[69] Samadi Z, Bambaeichi E, Valiani M, Shahshahan Z. Evaluation of changes in levels of Hyperandrogenism, hirsutism and menstrual regulation after a period of aquatic high intensity interval training in women with polycystic ovary syndrome. International Journal of Preventive Medicine. 2019;**10**:187. DOI: 10.4103/ijpvm.IJPVM_360_18

[70] Guzick DS, Wing R, Smith D, Berga SL, Winters SJ. Endocrine consequences of weight loss in obese, hyperandrogenic, anovulatory women. Fertility and Sterility. 1994;**61**(4): 598-604

[71] Pasquali R, Gambineri A, Cavazza C, Ibarra Gasparini D, Ciampaglia W, Cognigni GE, et al. Heterogeneity in the responsiveness to long-term lifestyle intervention and predictability in obese women with polycystic ovary syndrome. European Journal of Endocrinology. 2011;**164**(1):53-60. DOI: 10.1530/EJE-10-0692

[72] Dietz de Loos A, Jiskoot G, van den Berg-Emons R, Louwers Y, Beerthuizen A, van Busschbach J, et al. The effect of tailored short message service (SMS) on physical activity: Results from a three-component randomized controlled lifestyle intervention in women with PCOS. Journal of. Clinical Medicine. 2023;**12**(7): 2466. DOI: 10.3390/jcm12072466

[73] Redman LM, Elkind-Hirsch K, Ravussin E. Aerobic exercise in women with polycystic ovary syndrome improves ovarian morphology independent of changes in body composition. Fertility and Sterility. 2011; **95**(8):2696-2699. DOI: 10.1016/j.fertnstert.2011.01.137

[74] Lu KT, Ho YC, Chang CL, Lan KC, Wu CC, Su YT. Evaluation of bodily pain associated with polycystic ovary syndrome: A review of health-related quality of life and potential risk factors. Biomedicine. 2022;**10**(12):3197. DOI: 10.3390/biomedicines10123197

[75] Tasali E, Van Cauter E, Ehrmann DA. Polycystic ovary syndrome and obstructive sleep Apnea. Sleep Medicine Clinics. 2008;**3**(1):37-46. DOI: 10.1016/j.jsmc.2007.11.001

[76] Engmann L, Jin S, Sun F, Legro RS, Polotsky AJ, Hansen KR, et al. Racial and ethnic differences in the polycystic ovary syndrome metabolic phenotype. American Journal of Obstetrics and Gynecology. 2017;**216**(5):493.e1. DOI: 10.1016/j.ajog.2017.01.003

[77] Stanaway F, Cumming RG, Blyth F. Exclusions from clinical trials in Australia based on proficiency in English. The Medical Journal of Australia. 2017;**207**(1):36. DOI: 10.5694/mja16.01012

[78] Bruner B, Chad K, Chizen D. Effects of exercise and nutritional counseling in women with polycystic ovary syndrome. Applied Physiology, Nutrition, and Metabolism. 2006;**31**(4):384-391. DOI: 10.1139/h06-007

[79] Thomson RL, Buckley JD, Noakes M, Clifton PM, Norman RJ, Brinkworth GD. The effect of a hypocaloric diet with and without exercise training on body

composition, cardiometabolic risk profile, and reproductive function in overweight and obese women with polycystic ovary syndrome. The Journal of Clinical Endocrinology and Metabolism. 2008;**93**(9):3373-3380. DOI: 10.1210/jc.2008-0751

[80] Almenning I, Rieber-Mohn A, Lundgren KM, Shetelig Løvvik T, Garnæs KK, Moholdt T. Effects of high intensity interval training and strength training on metabolic, cardiovascular and hormonal outcomes in women with polycystic ovary syndrome: A pilot study. PLoS One. 2015;**10**(9): e0138793. DOI: 10.1371/journal.pone.0138793

[81] Nasiri M, Monazzami A, Alavimilani S, Asemi Z. The effect of high intensity intermittent and combined (resistant and endurance) trainings on some anthropometric indices and aerobic performance in women with polycystic ovary syndrome: A randomized controlled clinical trial study. International Journal of Fertility and Sterility. 2022;**16**(4): 268-274. DOI: 10.22074/ijfs.2022.551096.1279

[82] Rao M, Khan AA, Adnan QUA. Effects of high-intensity interval training and strength training on levels of testosterone and physical activity among women with polycystic ovary syndrome. Obstetrics and Gynecology Science. 2022;**65**(4):368-375. DOI: 10.5468/ogs.22002

[83] Turan V, Mutlu EK, Solmaz U, Ekin A, Tosun O, Tosun G, et al. Benefits of short-term structured exercise in non-overweight women with polycystic ovary syndrome: A prospective randomized controlled study. Journal of Physical Therapy Science. 2015;**27**(7): 2293-2297. DOI: 10.1589/jpts.27.2293

[84] Aubuchon M, Laughbaum N, Poetker A, Williams D, Thomas M. Supervised short-term nutrition and exercise promotes weight loss in overweight and obese patients with polycystic ovary syndrome. Fertility and Sterility. 2009;**91**(4):1336-1338. DOI: 10.1016/j.fertnstert.2008.03.028

[85] Nybacka Å, Carlström K, Ståhle A, Nyrén S, Hellström PM, Hirschberg AL. Randomized comparison of the influence of dietary management and/or physical exercise on ovarian function and metabolic parameters in overweight women with polycystic ovary syndrome. Fertility and Sterility. 2011;**96**(6): 1508-1513. DOI: 10.1016/j.fertnstert.2011.09.006

[86] Curi DD, Fonseca AM, Marcondes JA, Almeida JA, Bagnoli VR, Soares JM Jr, et al. Metformin versus lifestyle changes in treating women with polycystic ovary syndrome. Gynecological Endocrinology. 2012;**28**(3):182-185. DOI: 10.3109/09513590.2011.583957

[87] Aqdas A, Rafique S, Naeem E, Saleem N, Muneeb HN, Hamid MF, et al. Effects of resistance exercise on lipid profile and body mass index In women with poly cystic ovary syndrome: Effects of resistance exercise on women with poly cystic ovary syndrome. Pakistan BioMedical Journal. 2022;**2022**:109-113. DOI: 10.54393/pbmj.v5i4.367

[88] Zhang J, Si Q, Li J. Therapeutic effects of metformin and clomiphene in combination with lifestyle intervention on infertility in women with obese polycystic ovary syndrome. Pakistan Journal of Medical Science. 2017;**33**(1): 8-12. DOI: 10.12669/pjms.331.11764

[89] Lara LAS, Ramos FKP, Kogure GS, Costa RS, Silva de Sá MF, Ferriani RA, et al. Impact of physical resistance training on the sexual function of

women with polycystic ovary syndrome. The Journal of Sexual Medicine. 2015; **12**(7):1584-1590. DOI: 10.1111/jsm.12909

[90] Ramos FK, Lara LA, Kogure GS, Silva RC, Ferriani RA, Silva de Sá MF, et al. Quality of life in women with polycystic ovary syndrome after a program of resistance exercise training. Revista Brasileira de Ginecologia e Obstetrícia. 2016;**38**(7): 340-347

[91] Thomson RL, Buckley JD, Brinkworth GD. Perceived exercise barriers are reduced and benefits are improved with lifestyle modification in overweight and obese women with polycystic ovary syndrome: A randomised controlled trial. BMC Women's Health. 2016;**16**:14. DOI: 10.1186/s12905-016-0292-8

[92] Kogure GS, Miranda-Furtado CL, Pedroso DCC, Ribeiro VB, Eiras MC, Silva RC, et al. Effects of progressive resistance training on obesity indices in polycystic ovary syndrome and the relationship with telomere length. Journal of Physical Activity & Health. 2019;**16**(8):601-607. DOI: 10.1123/jpah.2018-0256

[93] Kogure GS, Silva RC, Miranda-Furtado CL, Ribeiro VB, Pedroso DCC, Melo AS, et al. Hyperandrogenism enhances muscle strength after progressive resistance training, independent of body composition, in women with polycystic ovary syndrome. Journal of Strength and Conditioning Research. 2018;**32**(9):2642-2651. DOI: 10.1519/JSC.0000000000002714

[94] Kogure GS, Miranda-Furtado CL, Silva RC, Melo AS, Ferriani RA, De Sá MF, et al. Resistance exercise impacts lean muscle mass in women with polycystic ovary syndrome. Medicine and Science in Sports and Exercise. 2016; **48**(4):589-598. DOI: 10.1249/MSS.0000000000000822

[95] Miranda-Furtado CL, Ramos FKP, Kogure GS, Santana-Lemos BA, Ferriani RA, Calado RT, et al. A nonrandomized trial of progressive resistance training intervention in women with polycystic ovary syndrome and its implications in telomere content. Reproductive Sciences. 2016;**23**(5): 644-654. DOI: 10.1177/1933719115611753

[96] Saremi A, Yaghoubi MS. Effect of resistance exercises with calcium consumption on level of anti-mullerian hormone and some metabolic indices in women with polycystic ovarian syndrome. The Iranian Journal of Obstetrics, Gynecology and Infertility. 2016;**18**(180):7-15. DOI: 10.22038/IJOGI.2016.6581

[97] Hosseini SA, Kazemi N, Shadmehri S, Jalili S, Ahmadi M. The effect of resistance training in water and land with vitamin D supplementation on anti-Mullerian hormone in women with polycystic ovary syndrome. Women's Health Bulletin. 2019;**6**(2):1-6. DOI: 10.5812/whb.84882

[98] Saeed A, Kemall F, Iqbal J, Sarwar R, Mustafa M, Tahir M. Effect of resistance exercise training program on quality of life in women with and without polycystic ovary syndrome; a cross sectional survey. Pakistan Journal of Medical & Health Sciences. 2022;**16**(7): 956. DOI: 10.53350/pjmhs22167956